A CHINESE-ENGLISH HANDBOOK OF
ACUPUNCTURE
AND MOXIBUSTION

汉英针灸治疗手册

谢金华 符文彬 叶苇\编著
司徒铃 教授\指导

江西科学技术出版社

序

　　谢金华氏和符文彬氏,广东针灸后起之秀,孜孜不倦,他们虚心向前辈学习,认真总结经验以形成自己的特色。作为中医学院的教师和作为一个临床医生,他们最了解学生以及医生的需求。《汉英针灸治疗手册》一书,由谢、符两位医生编著,它包括上下两篇,理论与实践相结合,中英合璧,别开生面,方便中外医生。

　　老朽有幸,得以先睹为快,并乐为之序。希望此书能为联合国提出的"二〇〇〇年,人人享有卫生保健"目标的实现作出贡献。

彭静山
序于沈阳　静思庐
一九九四年中秋月圆时

PREFACE

Dr. Xie Jinhua and Dr. Fu Wenbin, two acupuncturists in Guangdong province, have been diligently studying in the field of acupuncture and moxibustion for many years. They have learnt through theguidance of senior doctors and gradually developed their own techniques. As teachers in medical college and practioners in clinic, they are able to understand the needs of practioners and medical students. A Chinese-English Handbook of Acupuncture and Moxibustion, compiled by Dr. Xie and Dr. Fu, consists of two parts. It is the integration of theory and practical experience. As a bilingual book (Chinese-English), it will also serve the needs of many readers abroad.

It is my pleasure to be able to read this manuscript and to be asked to write the preface for this book. We hope that this book will help to accomplish of the aim, advocated by WHO: the possibility of attaining by all citizens of the world by the year 2000 a level of health that will permit them to lead a socially and economically productive life.

Peng Jinshan
in Jing Si Room, Shenyang
Oct. 1994

前　言

　　《汉英针灸治疗手册》作为一本针灸学的临床参考书，其编写目的很明确，即为针灸临床及临床教学提供一本简便实用的工具书。因此，它不求覆盖针灸学的各个方面。

　　书中所列各种疗法，许多已在其他一些针灸学参考书中提到。有些在临床上只是作为一种疾病的辅助性治疗手段，例如针灸治疗某些急症或一些外科疾病。因此，请读者注意。

　　本书编写过程中曾得到许多朋友的帮助、鼓励与支持，这些朋友的帮助、支持和鼓励使得该手册的出版成为可能。本书引用收集了许多针灸学的最新研究成果，书后所列的参考书目只是一些最主要的，其余未列者则在此一并致谢。

　　全书在编写过程中曾得到了司徒铃教授以及彭静山教授的精心指导，在此深表感谢。

　　由于编者的学术水平有限，缺点错误在所难免，欢迎批评指正。

编　者

一九九四年五月

FOREWORD

The Chinese-English Handbook of Acupuncture and Moxibustion is prepared as a convenient guide for acupuncturists in clinic.

The objective of the handbook is very clear, namely to provide a convenient guide for acupuncure practioners. It does not attempt to cover all aspects of acupuncture science. Many treatments of acupuncture and moxibustion compiled in this handbook have been recommended in many other books Some of these treatments, for example the acupuncture treatments of some medical emergencies and some surgical disorders, are practised only as supplementary treatments on many occassions in the clinic. It is advisable for the readers to pay attention to these aspects.

We are indebted to many people who helped to bring this handbook to publication. We are very grateful for the guidance of Professor Situ Ling and Professor Peng Jingshan, who have given necessary advice in the compilation of the handbook.

We have tried our best in compiling this handbook, but there may still be some errors. Any comment on the handbook and any suggestion for the further revision of this handbook will be much appreciated.

Compilers
May 1994

目 录
CONTENTS

上 篇　针灸学基本理论及常用技术
PART ONE　BASIC THEORY AND TECHNIQUES OF ACUPUNCTURE AND MOXIBUSTION

第一章　特定穴 ································· (3)
Chapter ane　Specific Points ································· (3)
　1.1　五输穴 ································· (3)
　1.1　Five-Shu Points ································· (3)
　1.2　十二脏腑募穴 ································· (6)
　1.2　The Front-Mu Points ································· (6)
　1.3　十二经原络穴 ································· (7)
　1.3　The Yuan-(Source) Points and Luo-(Connecting) Points of 12 Meridians ································· (8)
　1.4　八脉交会穴 ································· (9)
　1.4　The Eight Confluent Points of The Eight Extra-Meridians ······ (10)
　1.5　八会穴 ································· (11)
　1.5　The Eight Influential Points ································· (11)
　1.6　十六郄穴 ································· (12)
　1.6　The Sixteen Xi-(cleft) Points ································· (13)
　1.7　下合穴 ································· (14)
　1.7　The Lower He-(Sea) Points Pertaining to the Six-Fu Organs ········ (15)

第二章　头针疗法……………………………(16)
Chapter two　Scalp Acupuncture ……………(16)
   2.1　头针选穴原则………………………(16)
   2.1　Principles of Site Selection …………(16)
   2.2　操作方法……………………………(17)
   2.2　Method ………………………………(17)
   2.3　疗程…………………………………(18)
   2.3　Therapeutic Course …………………(18)
   2.4　刺激区的部位及主治作用…………(19)
   2.4　The Locations and Indications of Scalp Area ………(19)

第三章　耳针疗法……………………………(30)
Chapter three　Auricular Points Therapy ……(30)
   3.1　常用耳穴示意图……………………(30)
   3.1　Schematic Diagram of Distribution of Auricular Points ………(30)
   3.2　常用耳穴定位及主治………………(30)
   3.2　The Locations and Indications of Auriculars Points ………(30)

第四章　眼针疗法……………………………(51)
Chapter four　Eye Acupuncture ………………(51)
   4.1　眼针治疗的原理……………………(51)
   4.1　The Principle of Eye Acupuncture ……(51)
   4.2　眼针穴位分布及功效主治…………(54)
   4.2　The Location Functions and Indications of the Eye Acupoints ……………………………………………(54)
   4.3　眼针取穴原则………………………(57)
   4.3　Method of Selecting Eye Acupoints …(57)
   4.4　眼针配穴原则举例…………………(58)
   4.4　Examples of Eye Acupoints Treatment Prescriptions ………(58)
   4.5　眼针操作方法………………………(61)
   4.5　The Manipulation of Eye Acupuncture …(61)

第五章　子午流注针法………………………(62)

Chapter five Ziwu Liuzhu Acupuncture ················ (62)

- 5.1 天干地支的内容··································· (62)
- 5.1 Heavenly Stems and Earthly Branches ········· (62)
- 5.2 子午流注针法的组成······························· (62)
- 5.2 The Constitution of Ziwu Liuzhu Acupuncture ··· (62)
- 5.3 子午流注纳子法··································· (76)
- 5.3 The Method of Adopting Branches ·············· (76)
- 5.4 子午流注纳甲法··································· (80)
- 5.4 The Method of Adopting Stems ················· (80)

下篇 常见病的针灸治疗
PART TWO THE TREATMENT OF COMMON DISEASES

第一章 内科病症 ····································· (93)
Chapter one Internal Diseases ······················ (93)

- 1.1 中风·· (93)
- 1.1 Wind Stroke ······································ (93)
- 1.2 感冒·· (96)
- 1.2 Common Cold ···································· (96)
- 1.3 咳嗽·· (98)
- 1.3 Cough ··· (98)
- 1.4 哮喘··· (101)
- 1.4 Asthma ··· (101)
- 1.5 胃脘痛··· (104)
- 1.5 Epigastric Pain ··································· (104)
- 1.6 呕吐··· (107)
- 1.6 Vomiting ··· (107)
- 1.7 呃逆··· (109)
- 1.7 Hiccup ·· (109)
- 1.8 腹痛··· (111)

3

1.8	Abdominal Pain	(111)
1.9	泄泻	(113)
1.9	Diarrhoea	(113)
1.10	腹胀	(116)
1.10	Abdominal Distention	(116)
1.11	便秘	(118)
1.11	Constipation	(118)
1.12	脱肛	(120)
1.12	Prolapse of Rectum	(120)
1.13	水肿	(121)
1.13	Edema	(121)
1.14	遗尿	(123)
1.14	Nocturnal Enuresis	(123)
1.15	淋证	(124)
1.15	Urination Disturbance	(124)
1.16	癃闭	(127)
1.16	Retention of Urine	(127)
1.17	阳痿	(129)
1.17	Impotence	(129)
1.18	失眠	(131)
1.18	Insomnia	(131)
1.19	心悸	(133)
1.19	Palpitation	(133)
1.20	癫痫	(136)
1.20	Epilepsy	(136)
1.21	头晕	(139)
1.21	Dizziness	(139)
1.22	郁证	(141)
1.22	Melancholia	(141)
1.23	头痛	(144)
1.23	Headache	(144)

1.24 三叉神经痛 ………………………………………… (148)
1.24 Trigeminal Neuralgia ………………………………… (148)
1.25 周围性面瘫 ………………………………………… (151)
1.25 Peripheral Facial Paralysis ………………………… (151)
1.26 胁痛 ………………………………………………… (153)
1.26 Pain in Hypochondriac Region ……………………… (153)
1.27 腰痛 ………………………………………………… (155)
1.27 Low Back Pain ……………………………………… (155)
1.28 痹证 ………………………………………………… (158)
1.28 Bi-Syndrome ………………………………………… (158)
1.29 痿证 ………………………………………………… (162)
1.29 Wei-Syndrome ……………………………………… (162)

第二章 妇儿科病症 ………………………………………… (166)
Chapter two Gynecological and Pediatric Diseases ………… (166)

2.1 月经不调 …………………………………………… (166)
2.1 Irregular Menstruation ……………………………… (166)
2.2 痛经 ………………………………………………… (172)
2.2 Dysmenorrhea ……………………………………… (172)
2.3 闭经 ………………………………………………… (174)
2.3 Amenorrhea ………………………………………… (174)
2.4 崩漏 ………………………………………………… (176)
2.4 Uterine Bleeding …………………………………… (176)
2.5 带下病 ……………………………………………… (178)
2.5 Morbid Leukorrhea ………………………………… (178)
2.6 妊娠呕吐 …………………………………………… (180)
2.6 Morning Sickness …………………………………… (180)
2.7 乳汁不足 …………………………………………… (182)
2.7 Insufficient Lactation ……………………………… (182)
2.8 婴儿腹泻 …………………………………………… (184)
2.8 Infantile Diarrhoea ………………………………… (184)
2.9 小儿疳积 …………………………………………… (186)

| 2.9 | Infantile Malnutrition | (186) |

第三章　眼、耳、鼻、喉及外科诸症 …………………… (188)

Chapter three　External Diseases and Diseases of Eyes, Ears, Nose and Throat …………………………………… (188)

3.1	荨麻疹 ……………………………………	(188)
3.1	Urticaria …………………………………	(188)
3.2	带状疱疹 …………………………………	(190)
3.2	Herps Zoster ……………………………	(190)
3.3	耳聋、耳鸣 ………………………………	(191)
3.3	Deafness and Tinnitus …………………	(191)
3.4	目赤肿痛 …………………………………	(193)
3.4	Congestion, Swelling and Pain of Eye …	(193)
3.5	鼻渊 ………………………………………	(195)
3.5	Thick and Sticky Nasal Discharge ……	(195)
3.6	鼻衄 ………………………………………	(196)
3.6	Epistaxis …………………………………	(196)
3.7	牙痛 ………………………………………	(197)
3.7	Toothache ………………………………	(197)
3.8	咽喉痛 ……………………………………	(199)
3.8	Sore Throat ……………………………	(199)
3.9	视神经萎缩 ………………………………	(201)
3.9	Optic Atrophy …………………………	(201)

第四章　其他病症 …………………………………… (204)

Chapter four　Miscellaneous Diseases ………… (204)

4.1	粉刺 ………………………………………	(204)
4.1	Acne ……………………………………	(204)
4.2	肥胖症 ……………………………………	(207)
4.2	Obesity …………………………………	(207)
4.3	雀斑 ………………………………………	(210)
4.3	Freckle …………………………………	(210)

1.24	三叉神经痛	(148)
1.24	Trigeminal Neuralgia	(148)
1.25	周围性面瘫	(151)
1.25	Peripheral Facial Paralysis	(151)
1.26	胁痛	(153)
1.26	Pain in Hypochondriac Region	(153)
1.27	腰痛	(155)
1.27	Low Back Pain	(155)
1.28	痹证	(158)
1.28	Bi-Syndrome	(158)
1.29	痿证	(162)
1.29	Wei-Syndrome	(162)

第二章 妇儿科病症 (166)
Chapter two Gynecological and Pediatric Diseases (166)

2.1	月经不调	(166)
2.1	Irregular Menstruation	(166)
2.2	痛经	(172)
2.2	Dysmenorrhea	(172)
2.3	闭经	(174)
2.3	Amenorrhea	(174)
2.4	崩漏	(176)
2.4	Uterine Bleeding	(176)
2.5	带下病	(178)
2.5	Morbid Leukorrhea	(178)
2.6	妊娠呕吐	(180)
2.6	Morning Sickness	(180)
2.7	乳汁不足	(182)
2.7	Insufficient Lactation	(182)
2.8	婴儿腹泻	(184)
2.8	Infantile Diarrhoea	(184)
2.9	小儿疳积	(186)

2.9　Infantile Malnutrition ……………………………………（186）

第三章　眼、耳、鼻、喉及外科诸症…………………（188）
Chapter three　External Diseases and Diseases of Eyes, Ears, Nose and Throat ……………………………………………（188）

3.1　荨麻疹 ………………………………………………（188）
3.1　Urticaria ……………………………………………（188）
3.2　带状疱疹 ……………………………………………（190）
3.2　Herps Zoster ………………………………………（190）
3.3　耳聋、耳鸣 …………………………………………（191）
3.3　Deafness and Tinnitus ……………………………（191）
3.4　目赤肿痛 ……………………………………………（193）
3.4　Congestion, Swelling and Pain of Eye …………（193）
3.5　鼻渊 …………………………………………………（195）
3.5　Thick and Sticky Nasal Discharge ………………（195）
3.6　鼻衄 …………………………………………………（196）
3.6　Epistaxis ……………………………………………（196）
3.7　牙痛 …………………………………………………（197）
3.7　Toothache …………………………………………（197）
3.8　咽喉痛 ………………………………………………（199）
3.8　Sore Throat ………………………………………（199）
3.9　视神经萎缩 …………………………………………（201）
3.9　Optic Atrophy ……………………………………（201）

第四章　其他病症 ………………………………………（204）
Chapter four　Miscellaneous Diseases ……………………（204）

4.1　粉刺 …………………………………………………（204）
4.1　Acne ………………………………………………（204）
4.2　肥胖症 ………………………………………………（207）
4.2　Obesity ……………………………………………（207）
4.3　雀斑 …………………………………………………（210）
4.3　Freckle ……………………………………………（210）

4.4	美尼尔氏综合征	(212)
4.4	Meniere's Syndrome	(212)
4.5	高脂血症	(215)
4.5	Hyperlipemia	(215)
4.6	结肠激惹综合征	(218)
4.6	Irritable Colon Syndrome	(218)
4.7	前列腺炎	(221)
4.7	Prostatitis	(221)

第五章 急症处理 (224)
Chapter five The Treatment of Emergencies (224)

5.1	厥脱	(224)
5.1	Syncope	(224)
5.2	惊厥抽搐	(227)
5.2	Convulsions	(227)
5.3	高热昏迷	(228)
5.3	Coma Due to High Fever	(228)
5.4	溺水	(230)
5.4	Near-Drowning	(230)
5.5	急性一氧化碳中毒	(231)
5.5	Acute Carbon Monoxide Poisoning	(231)
5.6	高山反应	(232)
5.6	Altitude Stress	(232)
5.7	放射反应	(233)
5.7	Radioreactions	(233)
5.8	急性白血病	(235)
5.8	Acute Leukemia	(235)
5.9	心绞痛	(236)
5.9	Angina Pectoris	(236)
5.10	心肌梗塞	(237)
5.10	Myocardic Infarction	(237)
5.11	急性胆囊炎	(239)

5.11	Acute Cholecystitis	(239)
5.12	胆石症	(240)
5.12	Gallstone	(240)
5.13	胆道蛔虫症	(242)
5.13	Biliary Ascariasis	(242)
5.14	消化性溃疡急性穿孔	(243)
5.14	Acute Perforation of Peptic Ulcer Diseases	(243)
5.15	急性幽门梗阻	(245)
5.15	Acute Pylorochesis	(245)
5.16	急性肠梗阻	(246)
5.16	Acute Intestinal Obstruction	(246)
5.17	急性胰腺炎	(248)
5.17	Acute Pancreatitis	(248)
5.18	急性阑尾炎	(250)
5.18	Acute Appendicitis	(250)
5.19	肾绞痛	(252)
5.19	Renal Colic	(252)
5.20	滞产	(253)
5.20	Prolonged Labor	(253)
5.21	新生儿窒息	(254)
5.21	Asphyxia Neonatorum	(254)
5.22	急性湿疹	(256)
5.22	Acute Eczema	(256)
5.23	破伤风	(257)
5.23	Tetanus	(257)
5.24	急性睾丸炎及附睾炎	(258)
5.24	Acute Testitis and Epididymo-orchitis	(258)
5.25	食物中毒	(260)
5.25	Food Poisoning	(260)
5.26	输液反应	(261)
5.26	Anaphylatic Reactions in Transfusion	(261)

5.27 青霉素过敏反应 ……………………………………… (262)
5.27 Anaphylatic Reactions to Penicillins ……………… (262)

第六章 常用针灸处方 ……………………………………… (264)
Chapter six Commonly-Used Prescriptions of Acupuncture and Moxibustion ……………………………………………………… (264)

  6.1 闪腰类方 ……………………………………………… (264)
  6.1 Prescriptions for Lumbago ………………………… (264)
  6.2 止喘即效方 …………………………………………… (271)
  6.2 Prescriptions for the Attack of Asthma ………… (271)
  6.3 坐骨神经痛类方 ……………………………………… (275)
  6.3 Prescriptions for Sciatica ………………………… (275)
  6.4 膝痛类方 ……………………………………………… (279)
  6.4 Prescriptions for Knee Joints Pain ……………… (279)
  6.5 中风偏瘫类方 ………………………………………… (283)
  6.5 Prescriptions for Hemiplegia After Apoplexy …… (283)
  6.6 面瘫类方 ……………………………………………… (287)
  6.6 Prescriptions for Peripheral Facial Paralysis …… (287)
  6.7 呃逆类方 ……………………………………………… (291)
  6.7 Prescriptions for Hiccup …………………………… (291)
  6.8 胃痛类方 ……………………………………………… (295)
  6.8 Prescriptions for Stomachache …………………… (295)
  6.9 中暑类方 ……………………………………………… (297)
  6.9 Prescriptions for Sunstroke ……………………… (297)
  6.10 腹泻类方 …………………………………………… (299)
  6.10 Prescriptions for Diarrhoea ……………………… (299)
  6.11 便秘类方 …………………………………………… (302)
  6.11 Prescriptions for Constipation …………………… (302)
  6.12 心悸类方 …………………………………………… (305)
  6.12 Prescriptions for Palpitation …………………… (305)
  6.13 心痛类方 …………………………………………… (306)
  6.13 Prescriptions for Precordial Pain ……………… (306)

6.14	胁痛类方	(309)
6.14	Prescriptions for Hypochondriac Region Pain	(309)
6.15	失眠类方	(312)
6.15	Prescriptions for Insomnia	(312)
6.16	高血压头眩晕类方	(314)
6.16	Prescriptions for Dizziness due to Hypertension	(314)
6.17	头痛类方	(317)
6.17	Prescriptions for Headache	(317)
6.18	癫痫类方	(321)
6.18	Prescriptions for Epilepsy	(321)
6.19	消渴类方	(324)
6.19	Prescriptions for Diabetes	(324)
6.20	肩周炎类方	(326)
6.20	Prescriptions for Periarthritis of Shoulder	(326)
6.21	落枕类方	(329)
6.21	Prescriptions for Torticollis	(329)
6.22	痛经类方	(335)
6.22	Prescriptions for Dysmenorrhea	(335)
6.23	闭经类方	(339)
6.23	Prescriptions for Amenorrhea	(339)
6.24	崩漏类方	(341)
6.24	Prescriptions for Uterine Bleeding	(341)
6.25	乳腺增生类方	(345)
6.25	Prescriptions for Hyperplasia of Mammary Gland	(345)
6.26	胎位不正类方	(347)
6.26	Prescriptions for Abnormal Fetas Position	(347)
6.27	遗尿类方	(348)
6.27	Prescriptions for Enuresis	(348)
6.28	牙痛类方	(351)
6.28	Prescriptions for Toothache	(351)
6.29	咽喉肿痛类方	(354)

6.29	Prescriptions for Laryngopharyngitis	(354)
6.30	痤疮类方	(356)
6.30	Prescriptions for Acne	(356)
6.31	痹证类方	(358)
6.31	Prescriptions for Bi-Syndrome	(358)
6.32	面肌痉挛类方	(361)
6.32	Prescriptions for Muscular Spasm of Face	(361)
6.33	咳嗽类方	(363)
6.33	Prescriptions for Cough	(363)
6.34	感冒类方	(365)
6.34	Prescriptions for Common Cold	(365)
6.35	肥胖类方	(367)
6.35	Prescriptions for Obesity	(367)
6.36	戒毒、戒烟、戒酒类方	(369)
6.36	Prescriptions for Quiting Smoking, the Treatment of Drug-Addict and Alcohol Dependence	(369)
6.37	瘾疹类方	(371)
6.37	Prescriptions for Urticaria	(371)
6.38	痔疮类方	(375)
6.38	Prescriptions for Hemorrhoid	(375)
6.39	保健类方	(377)
6.39	Prescriptions for Health Preserving	(377)
6.40	胆绞痛类方	(379)
6.40	Prescriptions for Biliary Colic	(379)
6.41	肾绞痛类方	(381)
6.41	Prescriptions for the Renal Colic	(381)
6.42	三叉神经痛类方	(383)
6.42	Prescriptions for Trigeminal Neuralgia	(383)
6.43	内耳眩晕类方	(384)
6.43	Prescriptions for Auditory Vertigo	(384)
6.44	足跟痛类方	(386)

6.44　Prescriptions for Heel Pain ·· (386)
6.45　颈椎病类方 ·· (388)
6.45　Prescriptions for Cervical Spondylopathy ······················ (388)
6.46　治癣类方 ·· (390)
6.46　Prescriptions for Treatment of Tinea ···························· (390)
6.47　治牛皮癣类方 ·· (392)
6.47　Prescriptions for Psoriasis ·· (392)
6.48　麦粒肿类方 ·· (393)
6.48　Prescriptions for Hordeolum ······································· (393)
6.49　目赤肿痛类方 ·· (396)
6.49　Prescriptions for Redish, Painful and Swollen Eye ········· (396)
6.50　造血系统疾病类方 ·· (398)
6.50　Prescriptions for Disorders in Hematopoietic System ······ (398)
6.51　肿瘤类方 ·· (399)
6.51　Prescriptions for the Treatment of Tumor ······················ (399)

附录Ⅰ　　针灸穴位索引表 ································ (402)
Appendix one　Cross Index of Acupoints ······················ (402)
附录Ⅱ　　经外奇穴的定位 ································ (419)
Appendix two　The Locations of Extra-acupoints ············· (419)
附录Ⅲ　　参考文献 ·· (429)
Appendix three　The Biliography ································· (429)

上篇
针灸学基本理论
及常用技术

PART ONE
BASIC THEORY AND TECHNIQUES OF ACUPUNCTURRE AND MOXIBUSTION

第一章 特定穴
CHAPTER ONE SPECIFIC POINTS

1.1 五输穴
1.1 Five-shu Points

阴经五输穴表

五输 阴经	井(木)	荥(火)	输(土)	经(金)	合(水)
肺 手太阴	少商	鱼际	太渊	经渠	尺泽
心包 手厥阴	中冲	劳宫	大陵	间使	曲泽
心 手少阴	少冲	少府	神门	灵道	少海
脾 足太阴	隐白	大都	太白	商丘	阴陵泉
肝 足厥阴	大敦	行间	太冲	中封	曲泉
肾 足少阴	涌泉	然谷	太溪	复溜	阴谷

Table of Five-*SHU* Points of the Yin Meridians

Five *Shu* Points \ Channel	*Jing-* (Well) (Wood)	*Ying-* (Spring) (Fire)	*Shu-* (Stream) (Earth)	*Jing-* (River) (Metal)	*He-* (Sea) (Water)
Lung Hand-*Taiyin*	Shaoshang (LU11)	Yuji (LU10)	Taiyuan (LU9)	Jingqu (LU8)	Chize (LU5)
Pericardium Hand-*Jueyin*	Zhongchong (PC9)	Laogong (PC8)	Daling (PC7)	Jianshi (PC5)	Quze (PC3)
Heart Hand-*Shaoyin*	Shaochong (HT9)	Shaofu (HT8)	Shenmen (HT7)	Lingdao (HT4)	Shaohai (HT3)
Spleen Foot-*Taiyin*	Yinbai (SP1)	Dadu (SP2)	Taibai (SP3)	Shangqiu (SP5)	Yinlingquan (SP9)
Liver Foot-*Jueyin*	Dadun (LR1)	Xingjian (LR2)	Taichong (LR3)	Zhong-feng (LR4)	Ququan (LR8)
Kidney Foot-*Shaoyin*	Yongquan (KI1)	Rangu (KI2)	Taixi (KI3)	Fuliu (KI7)	Yingu (KI10)

阳经五输穴表

阳经 \ 五输	井(金)	荥(水)	输(木)	经(火)	合(土)
大肠　手阳明	商阳	二间	三间	阳溪	曲池
三焦　手少阳	关冲	液门	中渚	支沟	天井
小肠　手太阳	少泽	前谷	后溪	阳谷	小海
胃　　足阳明	厉兑	内庭	陷谷	解溪	足三里
胆　　足少阳	足窍阴	侠溪	足临泣	阳辅	阳陵泉
膀胱　足太阳	至阴	足通谷	束骨	昆仑	委中

Table The Five-*SHU* Points of the Yang Meridians

Five Shu Points / Channel	Jing- (Well) (Metal)	Ying- (Spring) (Water)	Shu- (Stream) (Wood)	Jing- (River) (Fire)	He- (Sea) (Earth)
Large Intestine Hand- *Rangming*	Shangyang (LI1)	Erjian (LI2)	Sanjian (LI3)	Yangxi (LI5)	Quchi (LI11)
Sanjiao Hand- *Shaoyang*	Guanchong (SJ1)	Yemen (SJ2)	Zhongzhu (SJ3)	Zhigou (SJ6)	Tianjing (SJ10)
Small Intestine Hand- *Taiyang*	Shaoze (SI1)	Qiangu (SI2)	Houxi (SI3)	Yanggu (SI5)	Xiaohai (SI8)
Stomach Foot- *Rangming*	Lidui (ST45)	Neiting (ST44)	Xiangu (ST43)	Jiexi (ST41)	Zusanli (ST36)
Gallbladder Foot-*Shaoyang*	Zuqiaoyin (GB44)	Xiaxi (GB43)	Zulinqi (GB41)	Yangfu (GB38)	Yanglingquar (GB34)
Bladder Foot- *Taiyang*	Zhiyin (BL67)	Zutonggu (BL66)	Shugu (BL65)	Kunlun (BL60)	Weizhong (BL40)

1.2 十二脏腑募穴

募穴	中府	膻中	巨阙	期门	章门	京门
脏	肺	心包	心	肝	脾	肾
募穴	中脘	日月	中极	天枢	石门	关元
腑	胃	胆	膀胱	大肠	三焦	小肠

1.2 The Front-Mu Points

Internal Organs   Front-mu Points

Lung   Zhongfu(LU 1)

Porioardium   Tanzhong(RN 17)

Heart   Juque(RN 14)

Liver   Qimen(LI-14)

Gallbladder   Riyue(GB 24)

Spleen	Zhangmem(LR 13)
Stomach	Zhongwan(RN 12)
Sanjiao	Shimen(RN 5)
Kidney	Jingmen(GB 25)
Large Intestine	Tianshu(SJ 25)
Small Intestine	Guanyuan(RN 4)
Bladder	Zhongji(RN 3)

1.3 十二经原络穴

经　脉	原穴	络穴	经　脉	原穴	络穴
手太阴肺	太渊	列缺	手阳明大肠	合谷	偏历
手厥阴心包	大陵	内关	手少阳三焦	阳池	外关
手少阴心	神门	通里	手太阳小肠	腕骨	支正
足太阴脾	太白	公孙	足阳明胃	冲阳	丰隆
足厥阴肝	太冲	蠡沟	足少阳胆	丘墟	光明
足少阴肾	太溪	大钟	足太阳膀胱	京骨	飞扬

1.3 The Yuan-(Source) Points and Luo-(Connecting) Points of 12 Meridians

Meridians	Luo-Connecting Points	Yuan-Source Points
Lung Meridian of Hand Taiyin	Lieque (LU 7)	Taiyuan (LI 9)
Large Intestine Meridian of Hand Yangming	Pianli (LI 6)	Hegu (LI 4)
Stomach Meridian of Foot Yangming	Fenglong (ST 40)	Chongyang (ST 42)
Spleen Meridian of Foot Taiyin	Gongsun (SP 4)	Taibai (SP 3)
Heart Meridian of Hand Shaoyin	Tongli (HT 5)	Shenmen (HT 7)
Small Intestine Meridian of Hand Taiyang	Zhizheng (SI 7)	Wangu (SI 4)
Bladder Meridian of Foot Taiyang	Feiyang (BL 58)	Jinggu (BL 64)
Kidney Meridian of Foot Shaoyin	Dazhong (KI 4)	Taixi (KI 3)
Pericardium Meridian of Hand Jueyin	Neiguan (PC 6)	Daling (PC 7)
Sanjiao Meridian of Hand Shaoyang	Waiguan (SJ 5)	Yangchi (SJ 4)

Gallbladder Meridian of Foot Shaoyang	Guangming (GB 37)	Qiuxu (GB 40)
Liver Meridian of Foot Jueyin	Ligou (LI 5)	Taichong (LI 3)

Note: The Luo-Connecting point of Ren Meridian is Jiuwei (RN 15), of Du Meridian, Changqian (DU 1), and the Major Luo Connecting of Spleen is Dabao (SP 21).

1.4 八脉交会穴

穴　位	所通脉	合　于
内关	阴维	心、胸、胃
公孙	冲脉	
后溪	督脉	颈、肩、背 目内眦
申脉	阳跷	
外关	阳维	耳后、颊、目外眦
足临泣	带脉	
列缺	任脉	咽喉、胸膈、肺系
照海	阴跷	

1.4 The Eight Confluent Points of the Eight Extra Meridians

Confluent Point	Extra Meridian	Indications
Neiguan (PC 6)	Yinwei	heart, chest, stomach
Gongsun (SP 4)	Chong	
Houxi (SI 3)	Du	neck, shoulder, back inner canthus
Shenmai (BL 62)	Yangqiao	
Waiguan (SJ 5)	Yangwei	retroauricle, cheek, outer canthus
Zuliqi (GB 41)	Dai	
Lieque (LI 7)	Ren	throat, chest, lung
Zhaohai (KI 6)	Yinqiao	

1.5 八会穴

脏会章门　　筋会阳陵
腑会中脘　　脉会太渊
气会膻中　　骨会大杼
血会膈俞　　髓会绝骨

1.5 The Eight Influential Points

Tissue	Influential Points
Zang organs	Zhangmen(LR 13)
Fu organs	Zhongwan(RN 12)
Qi	Tanzhong(RN 17)
Blood	Geshu(BL 17)
Tendon	Yanglingquan(GB 34)
Vessels	Taiyuan(LU 9)
Bone	Dazhu(BL 11)
Marrow	Juegu(GB 39)

1.6 十六郄穴

经　　脉	郄　　穴		经　　脉
手太阴肺经	孔最	水泉	足少阴肾经
手厥阴心包经	郄门	梁丘	足阳明胃经
手少阴心经	阴郄	外丘	足少阳胆经
手阳明大肠经	温溜	金门	足太阳膀胱经
手少阳三焦经	会宗	筑宾	阴维脉
手太阳小肠经	养老	阳交	阳维脉
足太阴脾经	地机	交信	阴跷脉
足厥阴肝经	中都	跗阳	阳跷脉

1.6 The Sixteen Xi-(cleft) Points

	Meridian	Xi-(Cleft) Point
Three Yin Meridians of Hand	Lung Meridian of Hand Taiyin	Kongzui(Lu 6)
	Pericardium Meridian of Hand Jueyin	Ximen(PC 4)
	Heart Meridian oHando of Hand Shaoyin	Yinxi(HT 6)
Three Yang meridians of Foot	Large Intestine Meridian of Hand Yangming	Wenliu(LI 7)
	Sanjiao Meridian of Hand Shaoyang	Huizong(SJ 7)
	Small Intestine Meridian of Hand Taiyang	Yanglao(SI 6)
Three Yang Meridians of Foot	Stomach Meridian of Foot Yangming	Liangqiu(ST 34)
	Gallbladder Meridian of Foot Shaoyang	Waiqiu(GB 36)
	Bladder Meridian of Foot Taiyang	Jinmen(BL 63)

Three Yin	Spleen Meridian of foot Taiyin	Diji(SP 8)
Meridians	Liver Meridian of Foot Jueyin	Zhongdu(LR 6)
of Hand	Kidney Meridian of Foot Shaoyin	Shuiquan(KI 5)

Extra	Yangqiao Meridian	Fuyang(BL 59)
Meridians	Yinqiao Meridian	Jiaoxin(KI 8)
	Yangwei Meridian	Yangjiao(G 35)
	Yinwei Meridian	Zhubin(KI 9)

1.7 下合穴

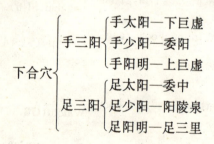

1.7 The Lower He-(Sea) Poinsts Pertaining to the Six-Fu Organs

Six Fu-Organs	Lower He-(Sea) Point
Stomach	Zusanli (ST 36)
Large intestine	ShangJuxu (ST 37)
Small intestine	Xiajuxu (XT 39)
Gallbladder	Yanglingquan (GB 34)
Bladder	Weizhong (BL 40)
Sanjiao	Weiyang (BL 39)

第二章 头针疗法
CHAPTER TWO SCALP ACUPUNCTURE

2.1 头针选穴原则
2.1 Principles of Site Selection

单侧肢体疾病,选用对侧刺激区;双侧肢体疾病,选用双侧刺激区;内脏、全身疾病或不易区别左右的疾病,可双侧取穴。一般根据疾病选用相应的刺激区,并可选用有关刺激区配合治疗,如下肢瘫痪可选用下肢运动区配足运感区。

For diseases affecting only one limb, a site is selected on the contralateral side of the head. Diseases affecting the limbs bilaterally are treated by stimulating sites on both sides of the head. Diseases of the internal organs or those which are systemic in nature, or those illnesses which are difficult to distinguish as being on one side or the other are treated by stimulating sites on both sides of the head. For instance, when treating paralysis of the lower limb, the principal site is the lower limb and trunk area in the motor area, supplemented by leg motor and sensory area.

2.2 操作方法
2.2 Method

明确诊断,选定刺激区,取得病员合作。病员取坐位或卧位,分开头发,常规消毒,选用 26～30 号 1.5～2.5 寸长的不锈钢毫针。

Diagnosing the diseases, selecting the area to be stimulated and asking the cooperation of patients. Expose the scalp and clean with alcohol. Usually 26—30, 1.5 to 2.5 cun in length stainless steel filiform needles are used.

2.2.1 快速进针
2.2.1 Swift Insertion

针尖与头皮呈 30°左右夹角,快速刺入皮下,然后沿刺激区快速推进(不捻转)到相应的深(长)度(或用捻转法进针)。

The needle is inserted in an angle of 30° to the scalp swiftly, Then inserted further along the area stimulated to be (not rorating) to requisite portion. (or inserting the needle with Twirling method)

2.2.2 快速捻转
2.2.2 Rapid Twirling

进针以后,使针体来回快速旋转(200 次/分)左右,捻转持续约 0.5～1 分钟,然后静留针 5～10 分钟重复捻转,用同样的方法再捻转两次,即可起针。也可用电针代替手捻进行治疗,据报道电针刺激头皮相应刺激区,治疗脑血管意外后遗症偏瘫的疗效与手法捻转的疗效相同。

Once the needle is in place, it should be twirled 200 times per minute. Twirling may be continued for 0.5 to 1 minute after which the needle is left in place for 5 to 10 minutes, then twirled again.

After repeating this procedure twice, the needle is withdrawn. The hand—twirling can be replaced with electric stimulation. It is reported that the electric stimulation in cooresponding scalp area obtains same effectiveness as manual—twirling dose in the treatment of hemiplegia caused by CVA.

2.2.3 起针方法
2.2.3 Withdrawn Method

如针下无沉紧感,可快速抽拔出针,也可缓慢出针,起针后必须以消毒干棉球按压针孔片刻,以防出血。

The needle can be withdrawn swiftly or slowly. A cotton ball may be pressed against the puncture to prevent bleeding.

2.3 疗程
2.3 Therapeutic Course

隔日或每日针治一次,10~15次为一个疗程。隔5~7天后继续下一疗程。

The treatment is given once every or every other day. A course consists of ten to fifteen treatments. After 5 to 7 days recess, continue next course.

2.4 刺激区的部位及主治作用
2.4 The Location and Indication of Scalp Area

2.4.1 标定线和运动区定位
2.4.1 Lines of Measurement and Motor Area Measure

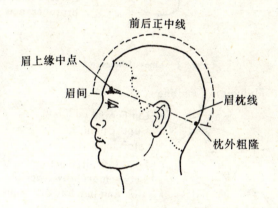

图 2.1 标定线

图 2.2 运动区定位

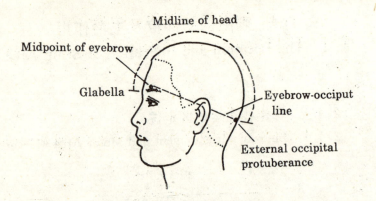

Fig2.1 Lines of Measurement

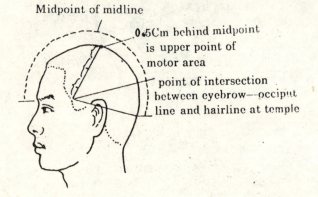

Fig2.2 Motor Area Measurements

2.4.2 侧面刺激区和顶面刺激区
2.4.2 Stimulation Areas Side View and Top View

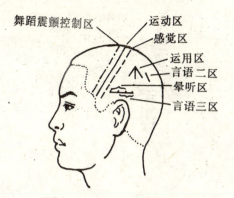

图 2.3 侧面刺激区

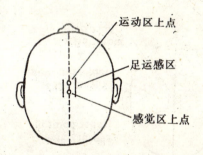

图 2.4 顶面刺激区

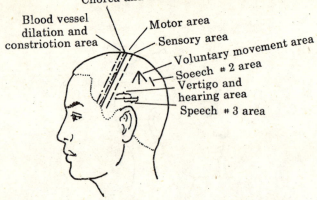

Fig2.3 Simulation Areas—Side View

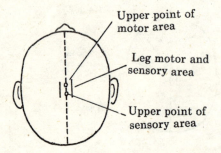

Fig2.4 Stimulation Areas—Top View

2.4.3 后面刺激区及前面刺激区
2.4.3 Stimulation Areas Back View and Front View

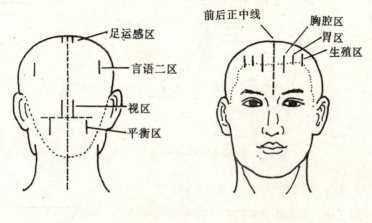

图 2.5 后面刺激区   图 2.6 前面刺激区

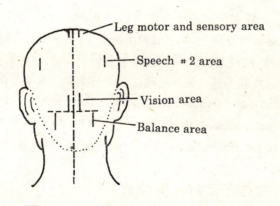

Fig2.5 Stimulation Areas—Back View

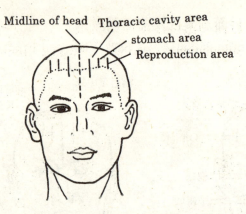

Fig2.6 Simulation Areas—Front View

2.4.4 刺激区部位及主治作用
2.4.4 Locations and Indications of the Areas

〔运动区〕

Motor area

部位:上点在前后正中线中点往后 0.5cm 处;下点在眉枕线和鬓角发际前缘相交处。如果鬓角不明显,可以从颧弓上缘中点向上引垂直线,此线与眉枕线交叉处向前移 0.5cm 为运动区下点。上下两点连线即为运动区。运动区又可分为上、中、下三部分。

Locatin: A line starting from a point 0.5 cm posterior to midpoint of midline and stretching diagonally across the head to a point at the intersection of the zygomatic arch (superior margin) with the hairline at the temple.

(1)下肢、躯干运动区:运动区的上 1/5;

(1)Lower limb and trunk area: Upper fifth of motor area line.

(2)面运动区(语言一区):运动区的下 2/5;

24

(2)Facial area (including speech No.1): Lower two fifths of motor area line.

(3)上肢运动区:运动区的中2/5。

(3)Upper limb area: Second and third fifths of motor area line.

主治:

Indications:

(1)下肢躯干运动区:对侧下肢、躯干部瘫痪;

(1)Lower limb and trunk area: Paralysis of lower limb (opposite side)

(2)面运动区:对侧中枢性面神经瘫痪,运动性失语、流涎、发音障碍;

(2)Facial area: Upper motor neuron paralysis of face (opposite side), motor aphasia, dribbling saliva, impaired speech.

(3)上肢运动区:对侧上肢瘫痪。

(3)Upper limb area: Paralysis of upper limb (opposite side).

〔感觉区〕

SENSORY AREA

部位:运动区向后移1.5厘米的平行线。本区分为上中下三部分。

Location: A line parallel and 1.5 cm posterior to the motor line.

(1)上部:感觉区的上1/5,为下肢、头、躯干感觉区;

(1)Lower limb、head and trunk area: Upper fifth of sensory area line

(2)中部:感觉区的中2/5,为上肢感觉区;

(2)Upper limb area: Second and third fifths of sensory area line.

(3)下部:感觉区的下2/5,为面感觉区。

(3)Facial area: Lower two fifths of sensory area line.

主治:

Indications:

(1)上部：对侧腰腿痛、麻木、感觉异常、后头、颈项疼痛，颈强、头晕、耳鸣；

(1) Lower limb, head and trunk area: Low back pain (opposite side), numbness or paresthesia in that area, occipital headache, stiff neck, vertigo and tinnitus.

(2)中部：对侧上肢疼痛、麻木、感觉异常；

(2) Upper limb area: Pain, numbness or other paresthesia of upper limb (opposite side)

(3)下部：对侧偏头痛、三叉神经痛、牙痛、颞颌关节炎。

(3) Facial area: Migraine headache, trigeminal e neuralgia, toothache (opposite side), arthritis of the e temporomandibular joint.

〔足运感区〕

LEG MOTOR AND SENSORY AREA

部位：前后正中线中点旁开左右各 1cm，向后引 3cm 长，平行于正中线。

Location: Parallel with midline of head, 1 cm beside midpoint (bilaterally), about 3 cm long.

主治：对侧下肢瘫痪、疼痛、麻木、急性腰扭伤、夜尿、皮质性多尿、子宫下垂等。

Indications: Paralysis, Pain, or numbness of lower limb, acute lower back sprain, nocturnal urination, prolapsed uterus.

〔舞蹈震颤控制区〕

CHOREA AND TREMOR CONTROL AREA

部位：运动区向前移 1.5cm 的平行线。

Location: Parallel with and 1.5cm anterior to motor area line.

主治：舞蹈病、震颤麻痹综合征。

Indications: Syndenham's chorea, tremors, palsy, and related syndromes.

〔晕听区〕

VERTIGO AND HEARING AREA

部位:从耳尖直上1.5cm处,向前及向后各引2cm的水平线,总长4cm。

Location: Horizontal line 1.5cm above and centered on the apx of ear, 4cm in length.

主治:眩晕、耳鸣、听力降低、美尼尔氏综合征。

Indications: Tinnitus, vertigo, diminished hearing, Menier's syndrome.

〔言语二区〕

SPEECH 2 AREA

部位:从顶骨结节后下方2cm处为起点引一平行于前后正中线的直线,向下取3cm长直线。

Location: Vertical line 2 cm beside tuber parietale on back of the head, 3 cm in length.

主治:命名性失语。

Indications: Nominal aphasia.

〔言语三区〕

SPEECH 3 AREA

部位:晕听区中点向后引4cm长的水平线。

Locations: Overlaps vertigo and hearing area at midpoint and continues 4 cm posteriorly.

主治:感觉性失语。

Indications: Receptive aphasia.

〔运用区〕

VOLUNTARY MOVEMENT AREA

部位:从顶骨结节起分别引一垂直线和与该线夹角为40度的

前后两线,长度均为 3cm。

Location: With the tuber parietale orgin, three needles can be inserted inferiorly, anteriorly and posteriorly to a length of 3 cm. Between them, the 3 lines will form a 40 degree angle.

主治:失用症。

Indication: Apraxia

〔视区〕

VISION AREA

部位:在前后正中线的后点旁开 1cm 处的枕外粗隆,向上引平行于前后正中线的 4cm 长的直线。

Location: One cm lateral to external occipital protuberance, parallel to midline of head, 4 cm in length extending upward.

主治:皮层性视力障碍。

Indications: Cortical Blindness.

〔平衡区〕

BALANCE AREA

部位:在前后正中线的后点旁开 3.5cm 处的枕外粗隆,向下引平行于前后正中线的 4cm 长的直线。

Location: Three cm lateral to the external occipital protuberance, parallel to midline of head, 4 cm in length, extending downward.

主治:小脑疾病引起的共济失调。

Indication: Loss of balance due to cerebellar disorders.

〔胃区〕

STOMACH AREA

部位:从瞳孔直上的发际为起点,向上引平行于前后正中线的 2cm 长的直线。

Location: Beginning at the hairline directly above pupil of eye, parallel with midline of head, 2 cm in length extending posteriorly.

主治：上腹部不适，胃痛。

Indication: Discomfort in upper abdomen.

〔胸腔区〕

THROACIC CAVITY AREA

部位：在胃区与前后正中线之间，发际上下各引 2cm 长的直线。

Location: Midway between and parallel with stomach area and midline of head, bilaterally, 2 cm in length.

主治：哮喘、胸痛、阵发性室上性心动过速。

Indications: Asthma, chest pain, intermittent supraventricular tachycardia.

〔生殖区〕

REPRODUCTION AREA

部位：从额角处向上引平行于前后正中线的 2cm 长的直线。

Location: Parallel and lateral to the stomach area at a distance equal to that between stomach and the thoracic cavity areas, 2 cm in length.

主治：功能性子宫出血，子宫脱垂（与足运感区合用）。

Indications: Abnormal utering bleeding, combined with leg motor area for prolapsed uterus.

第三章 耳针疗法
CHAPTER THREE AURICULAR POINTS THERAPY

3.1 常用耳穴示意图
3.1 Schematic Diagram of Distribution of Auricular Points

3.2 常用耳穴定位及主治
3.2 The Loctions and Indications of Auricular Points

3.2.1 耳轮脚及耳轮部
3.2.1 Helix and Helix Crus

3.2.1.1 耳中(膈)
3.2.1.1 Middle Ear (Diaphragm)
部位:在耳轮脚上。
Locations:Helix crus.
主治:呃逆,黄疸,消化不良,皮肤瘙痒。
Indications:Hiccup, jaundice, symptoms and disases of digestive

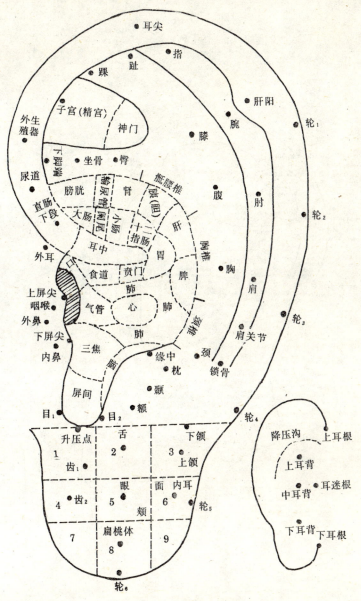

图 3.1 常用耳穴示意图

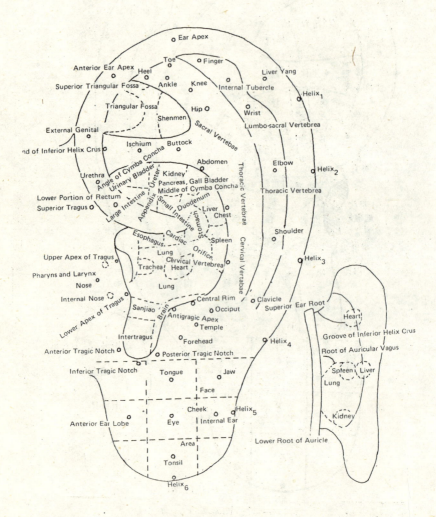

Fig 3.1　Schematic Diagram of Distribution of Anricular Points

system and skin itching.

3.2.1.2 直肠下段
3.2.1.2 Lower Portion of Rectum

部位:在与大肠穴同水平的耳轮处。

Location: On the end of helix approximate at the same level to large intestine point.

主治:便秘,痢疾,脱肛,痔疾。

Indications: Constipation, anus prolapse, external and internal hemarrhoids, tenesmus.

3.2.1.3 尿道
3.2.1.3 Urethra

部位:在对耳轮下脚下缘相平的耳轮处。

Location: On the helix at level with the lower border of inferior antihelix crus.

主治:尿频,尿急,尿痛,遗尿,尿潴留。

Indications: Enuresis, frequent, urgent and painful urination, retention of urine.

3.2.1.4 外生殖器
3.2.1.4 Extenal Genitalia

部位:在对耳轮下脚上缘相平的耳轮处。

Location: On helix at level with the upper border of inferior antihelix crus.

主治:阳痿,外生殖器炎症,会阴部湿疹。

Indications: Inflammation of external genital organs, eczema of the perineum, impotence.

3.2.1.5 耳尖
3.2.1.5 Ear Apex

部位:将耳轮向耳屏对折时,耳廓上尖端处。

Location: At the tip of auricle and superior to helix when folded towards tragus.

主治:发热,高血压,目赤肿痛,麦粒肿。

Indications: Fever, hypertension, conjunctivitis, hordeolum.

3.2.1.6 肝阳
3.2.1.6 Liver Yang

部位:在耳轮结节处。

Location: At auricular tubercle.

主治:肝气郁结,肝阳上亢。

Indications: Liver energy stagnation, liver Yang preponderance.

3.2.1.7 轮$_{1-6}$
3.2.1.7 Helix$_{1-6}$

部位:自耳轮结节下缘至耳垂正中下缘分成五等分,共六点,自上而下依次为轮$_1$……轮$_6$。

Location: Region from lower border of auricular tubercle to midpoint of lower border of lobule is divided into five equal parts. The points marking the divisions are respectively Helix 1, Helix 2, Helix 3, Helix 4, Helix 5, Helix 6.

主治:发热,扁桃体炎,高血压。

Indications: Fever, tonsillitis and hypertension.

3.2.2 耳舟部
3.2.2 Scapha

3.2.2.1 手指
3.2.2.1 Finger

部位:在耳舟顶部。

Location: At the top of scapha.

主治：手指麻木疼痛等。

Indications：Pain and numbness of the fingers.

3.2.2.2 腕
3.2.2.2 Wrist

部位：在平耳轮结节突起处的耳舟部。

Location：In scapha, at the same level with the top of auricle tubercle.

主治：腕部扭伤，肿痛等。

Indications：Pain and dysfunction at corresponding area of the body, wrist sprain.

3.2.2.3 肘
3.2.2.3 Elbow

部位：在手指穴和锁骨穴之间。

Location：Midway between finger and clavicle points.

主治：肘痹。

Indications：Pain in elbow.

3.2.2.4 肩
3.2.2.4 Shoulder

部位：在肘与锁骨之间。

Location：Midway between elbow and clavicle.

主治：肩痹。

Indications：Pain at shoulder joint.

3.2.2.5 锁骨
3.2.2.5 Clavicle

部位：在轮屏切迹同水平线的耳舟部。

Location：On scapha at level with Helix-tragic notch.

主治：相应部位疼痛，肩周炎。

Indications：Pain at the corresponding area of body, peri-arthritis

35

of the shoulder.

3.2.3 对耳轮上脚部
3.2.3 Superior Antihelix Crus

3.2.3.1 趾
3.2.3.1 Toe
部位:在对耳轮上脚的外上角。
Location:Superior and lateral angle of superior antihelix crus.
主治:足趾麻木,疼痛。
Indications:Numbness and pain at toes.

3.2.3.2 踝
3.2.3.2 Ankle
部位:对耳轮上脚的内上角。
Location:Superior and medial angle of superior of antihelix crus.
主治:踝关节炎,踝部扭伤等。
Indications:Pain and dysfunction at ankle joint, ankle sprain.

3.2.3.3 膝
3.2.3.3 Knee
部位:在对耳轮上脚的起始部,与对耳轮下脚上缘同水平。
Location:At the beginning of superior antihelix crus, at the same level with the superior border of inferior antihelix crus.
主治:膝关节炎,膝关节痛。
Indications:Pain, sprain and arthritis of the knee joint.

3.2.4 对耳轮下脚部
3.2.4 Inferior antihelix Crus

3.2.4.1 臀

3.2.4.1 Hip
部位:对耳轮下脚外 1/2 处。
Location: At the lateral 1/2 of the inferior antihelix crus.
主治:坐骨神经痛。
Indications: Sciatica.

3.2.4.2 坐骨
3.2.4.2 Ischium
部位:在对耳轮下脚内 1/2 处。
Location: At medial 1/2 of the inferior antihelix crus.
主治:坐骨神经痛。
Indications: Sciatica.

3.2.4.3 下脚端(交感)
3.2.4.3 End of Inferior Antihelix Crus (Sympathetic Nerve)
部位:在对耳轮下脚端与耳轮内侧交界处。
Location: The terminal of inferior antihelix crus.
主治:内脏痛症,心悸,自汗,盗汗,植物神经功能失调。
Indications: Pain of internal organs, palpitation, spontaneous sweating, night sweating, functional disorders of autonomous nerve system.

3.2.5 对耳轮部
3.2.5 Antihelix

3.2.5.1 脊椎
3.2.5.1 Vertebrae
部位:对耳轮的耳腔缘。将从轮屏切迹到对耳轮上下脚分叉部的曲线三等分,自上而下,下 1/3 颈椎,中 1/3 胸椎,上 1/3 腰骶椎。
Location: A curved line from helixtragic notch to the branching

area of superior and inferior antihelix crus can be divided into 3 equal segments. The lower 1/3 of it is Cervical Vertebrae, the middle 1/3 Thoracic Vertebrae, and the upper 1/3 Lumbosacral Vertebrae.

主治:相应部位疾病。

Indications: Disorders at corresponding area.

3.2.5.2 颈
3.2.5.2 Neck

部位:在颈椎的耳甲腔侧。

Location: On the border of cavum conchae of Cervical Vertebrae.

主治:落枕,颈部扭伤。

Indications: Strained neck, wry neck, pain or dysfunction of the neck.

3.2.5.3 胸
3.2.5.3 Chest

部位:在胸椎的耳甲腔侧。

Location: On the border of cavum conchae of Thoracic Vertebrae.

主治:胸闷胸痛。

Indications: Pain and stuffiness of the chest.

3.2.5.4 腹
3.2.5.4 Abdomen

部位:在腰骶椎的耳甲腔侧。

Location: On the border of cavum conchae of Lumbosacral Vertebrae points.

主治:腹部或妇科疾病,腰痛。

Indications: Abdominal or gynecological diseases, lumbago.

3.2.6 三角窝部
3.2.6 Triangular Fossa

3.2.6.1 神门
3.2.6.1 Ear-Shenmen
部位:在三角窝的外三分之一处,对耳轮上下脚交叉之前。

Location: At bifurcating point between superior and inferior antihelix crus, and at the lateral 1/3 of triangular fossa.

主治:失眠,多梦,烦躁,炎症,哮喘,咳嗽,眩晕,荨麻疹。可镇静、镇痛。

Indications: Insomnia, dream disturbed sleep, restlessness, inflammation, asthma, cough, vertigo, urtcaria. With the actions of sadation. Effective on easing mind, relieving pain.

3.2.6.2 子宫(精宫)
3.2.6.2 Uterus (Seminal Palace)
部位:在三角窝耳轮内侧缘中点。

Location: In the triangular fossa and in the depression close to the midpoint of helix.

主治:妇科病证,阳痿。

Indications: Gynecological diseases and symptoms, impotence.

3.2.7 耳屏部
3.2.7 Tragus

3.2.7.1 鼻(外鼻)
3.2.7.1 Nose (External Nose)
部位:在耳屏外侧面中央。

Location: In the centre of lateral aspect of tragus.

主治:鼻疖,鼻炎。

Indications: Nose fruncles, rhinitis.

3.2.7.2 上屏尖

3.2.7.2 **Supratragic Apex**

部位:在耳屏上部隆起的尖端。

Location: At the tip of upper protuberance on border of tragus.

主治:炎症及疼痛性疾病。

Indications: Inflammation and pain.

3.2.7.3 下屏尖(肾上腺)

3.2.7.3 **Infratragic Apex (Adrenal)**

部位:在耳屏下部隆起的尖端。

Location: At the tip of lower tubercle on border of tragus.

主治:热证,痛证,低血压,过敏性疾病。

Indications: Heat-syndrome, pain. hypotension and allergic diseases.

3.2.7.4 咽喉

3.2.7.4 **Pharynx-Larynx**

部位:在耳屏内侧面的上 1/2 处。

Location: Upper half of medial aspect of tragus.

主治:咽喉肿痛,扁桃体炎。

Indications: Sore throat and tonsillitis.

3.2.7.5 内鼻

3.2.7.5 **Internal Nose**

部位:在耳屏内侧面的下 1/2 处。

Location: Lower half of medial aspect of tragus.

主治:感冒,鼻炎,其他鼻疾。

Indications: Rhinitis, common cold, and other nose diseases.

3.2.8 对耳屏部

3.2.8 Antitragus

3.2.8.1 平喘(腮腺)

3.2.8.1 Soothing Asthma(Parotid)

部位:在对耳屏的尖端。

Location: At the tip of antitragic.

主治:哮喘,咳嗽,痄腮及遗尿。

Indications: Asthma, cough, parotitis and enuresis.

3.2.8.2 缘中(脑点)

3.2.8.2 Middle Border (Brain)

部位:在对耳屏间与轮屏切迹间的中点。

Location: Midpoint between antitragic apex and helix-tragic notch.

主治:遗尿,崩漏,急惊风。

Indications: Enuresis, abnormal uterus bleeding and acute infantile convulsion.

3.2.8.3 枕

3.2.8.3 Occiput

部位:在对耳屏外侧面的后上方。

Location: At posterior superior corner of lateral aspect of antitragus.

主治:头晕,头痛,失眠等。

Indications: Dizziness, headache, insomnia and etc.

3.2.8.4 颞(太阳)

3.2.8.4 Temple (Taiyang)

部位:在对耳屏外侧面,枕与额穴之间。

Location: On antitragus between Forehead and Occiput.

主治:偏头痛。

Indications: Migraine.

3.2.8.5 额

3.2.8.5 **Forehead**

部位:在对耳屏外侧面的前下方。

Location: At anterior inferior corner of lateral aspect of antitragus.

主治:阳明头痛,头昏,失眠,眩晕。

Indications: Yangming headache, dizziness, insomnia and vertigo.

3.2.8.6 **脑(皮质下)**

3.2.8.6 **Brain (Subcortex)**

部位:在对耳屏的内侧面。

Location: On medial aspect of antitragus.

主治:智能发育不全,失眠,多梦,肾虚耳鸣。

Indications: Oligophrenia, insomnia, dream disturbed sleep and tinnitus due to kidney deficiency.

3.2.9 耳轮脚周围部
3.2.9 Periphery Helix Crus

3.2.9.1 **口**

3.2.9.1 **Mouth**

部位:外耳道口的上缘和后缘。

Location: Close to posterior and superior border of orifice of external auditory meatus.

主治:面瘫,口腔炎症。

Indications: Facial paralysis, inflammation of mouth.

3.2.9.2 **食道**

3.2.9.2 **Esophagus**

部位:耳轮脚下方内2/3处。

Location: At medial 2/3 of inferior aspect of helix crus.

主治:恶心,呕吐,吞咽困难。

Indications: Dysphagia and vomitting.

3.2.9.3 贲门

3.2.9.3 Cardiac Orifice

部位:在耳轮脚下方外 1/3 处。

Location: At the lateral 1/3 of inferior aspect of helix crus.

主治:恶心,呕吐。

Indications: Nausea and vomiting.

3.2.9.4 胃

3.2.9.4 Stomach

部位:在耳轮脚消失处。

Location: At area where helix crus terminates.

主治:胃痛,呃逆,呕吐,消化不良,胃溃疡,失眠。

Indications: Stomachache, hiccup, vomiting, indigestion, gastric ulcer and insomnia.

3.2.9.5 十二指肠

3.2.9.5 Duodenum

部位:在耳轮脚上方外 1/3 处。

Location: At lateral 1/3 of superior aspect of helix crus.

主治:胆道疾病,十二指肠溃疡,幽门痉挛。

Indications: Disorders of biliary duct, duodenal ulcer and pylorospasm.

3.2.9.6 小肠

3.2.9.6 Small Intestine

部位:在耳轮脚上方中 1/3 处。

Location: At middle 1/3 of superior aspect of helix crus.

主治:消化不良,心悸。

Indications: Indigestion and palpitation.

3.2.9.7 阑尾

3.2.9.7 Appendix
部位：在小肠与大肠穴之间。

Location: Between Small Intestine and Large Intestine.

主治：阑尾炎,腹泻。

Indication: Appendicitis and diarrhoea.

3.2.9.8 大肠
3.2.9.8 Large Intestine
部位：在耳轮脚上方内1/3处。

Location: At medial 1/3 of superior aspect of helix crus.

主治：痢疾,腹泻,便秘。

Indications: Dysentery, diarrhoea and constipation.

3.2.10 耳甲艇部
3.2.10 Cymba Conchae

3.2.10.1 肝
3.2.10.1 Liver
部位：在胃、十二指肠穴后方。

Location: At posterior aspect of Stomach and Duodenum.

主治：肝气郁滞,眼疾,下侧腹部疾患。

Indications: Liver energy stagnation, eye diseases and disorders of lateral-lower abdomen.

3.2.10.2 胰
3.2.10.2 Pancrease
部位：在肝、肾穴之间。

Location: Between Liver and Kidney.

主治：胆道疾患,胰腺炎,偏头痛,糖尿病。

Indications: Diseases and symptoms of bile duct, pancreasitis, migraine and diabetis mellitus.

3.2.10.3 肾
3.2.10.3 Kidney

部位:对耳轮下脚的下缘,小肠穴直上方。

Location: On the lower border of inferior antihelix crus, directly above Small Intestine.

主治:泌尿、生殖、妇科疾病,腰痛,耳鸣,失眠,眩晕,颈、腰椎肥大。

Indications: Diseases and symptoms of urinary, reproductive systems and gynocology, lumbago, tinnitus, insomnia, dizziness, hypertrophy of lumber and cervical vertebrae.

3.2.10.4 输尿管
3.2.10.4 Ureter

部位:在膀胱与肾穴之间。

Location: Between Kidney and Bladder points.

主治:输尿管结石绞痛。

Indications: Stone and colic pain of ureter.

3.2.10.5 膀胱
3.2.10.5 Bladder

部位:在对耳轮下脚的下缘,大肠穴直上方。

Location: On the lower border of inferior antihelix crus, directly above the Large Intestine point.

主治:膀胱炎,尿闭,遗尿。

Indications: Cystitis, enuresis and retention of urine.

3.2.11 耳甲腔部
3.2.11 Cavum Conchae

3.2.11.1 心

3.2.11.1 **Heart**

部位:在耳甲腔中心最凹陷处。

Location: In the central depression of cavum conchae.

主治:失眠,心悸,癔病,盗汗,心绞痛。

Indications: Insomnia, palpitation, hysteria, night sweating, angina pectoris and etc.

3.2.11.2 肺

3.2.11.2 **Lung**

部位:在心穴的上、下、外三面。

Location: Around the Heart point.

主治:呼吸系统疾病,皮肤病,感冒。

Indications: Disorders and diseases of respiratary system, skin diseases and common cold.

3.2.11.3 气管

3.2.11.3 **Trachea**

部位:在肺穴内,心与口穴之间。

Location: In the area of Lung point, between Mouth and Heart points.

主治:咳嗽,哮喘。

Indications: Cough and asthma.

3.2.11.4 脾

3.2.11.4 **Spleen**

部位:肝穴下方,在耳甲腔的外上方。

Location: Inferior to Liver point, at lateral and superior aspect of cavum conchae.

主治:腹泻,腹胀,慢性消化不良,口腔炎症,功能性子宫出血。

Indications: Diarrhoea abdominal distension, chronic indigestion, stamotitis, functional uterus bleeding and etc.

3.2.11.5 三焦
3.2.11.5 Sanjiao
部位:在屏间穴上方。

Location: Superior to Intertragus.

主治:便秘,浮肿。

Indications: Constipation and edema.

3.2.12 耳垂部
3.2.12 Ear Lobule

3.2.12.1 眼$_1$
3.2.12.1 Eye$_1$
部位:屏间切迹的外前下方。

Location: On lateral and anterior side of intertragic notch.

主治:青光眼,假性近视,其他眼疾。

Indications: Glaucoma, pseudomyopia, and other eye diseases.

3.2.12.2 升压点
3.2.12.2 Elevating Blood Pressure Point
部位:在屏间切迹下方。

Location: On the inferior aspect of intertragic notch.

主治:低血压。

Indications: Hypotension.

3.2.12.3 眼$_2$
3.2.12.3 Eye$_2$
部位:在屏间切迹外后下方。

Location: On lateral and inferior aspect of intertragic notch.

主治:屈光不正,外眼炎症。

Indications: Ametropia, external eye inflammation and etc.

3.2.12.4 面颊
3.2.12.4 Cheek

部位:在眼穴的后方。

Location: On the ear lobe, at posterior aspect of Eye point.

主治:面瘫及其他面部疾病。

Indications: Facial paralysis and other facial problems.

3.2.12.5 舌
3.2.12.5 Tongue

部位:在耳垂2区的上方。

Location: At the superior of 2nd section of lobule.

主治:舌肿痛。

Indications: Glossitis.

3.2.12.6 下颌
3.2.12.6 Jaw

部位:在耳垂3区的上方。

Location: At the superior of 3rd section of lobule.

主治:牙痛(上牙),下颌关节痛。

Indications: Toothache, submandibular arthritis and etc.

3.2.12.7 眼
3.2.12.7 Eye

部位:在耳垂五区中央。

Location: In the 5th section of ear lobe.

主治:急性结膜炎,电光性眼炎,近视及其他眼病。

Indications: Acute conjunctivitis, electric ophthalmia, myopia and other eye diseases.

3.2.12.8 内耳

3.2.12.8 Internal Ear
部位:在耳垂的6区。

Location: In the 6th section of the ear lobe.

主治:耳鸣,听力障碍,耳源性眩晕。

Indications: Tinnitus, impaired hearing, auditory vertigo and etc.

3.2.12.9 扁桃腺
3.2.12.9 Tonsil
部位:在耳垂的8区。

Location: In the 8th section of the ear lobe.

主治:急性扁桃体炎。

Indications: Acute tonsillitis.

3.2.13 耳廓背面部
3.2.13 Back Auricle

3.2.13.1 上耳根
3.2.13.1 Upper Root of Auricle
部位:在耳根的最上缘。

Location: At the upper border of the auricular root.

主治:头痛,腹痛,哮喘。

Indications: Headache, abdominal pain and asthma.

3.2.13.2 下耳根
3.2.13.2 Lower Root of Auricle
部位:耳垂与面颊相交的下缘。

Location: On the lower border of the juncture between the ear lobe and the cheek.

主治:头痛,牙痛,咽喉痛,哮喘。

Indications: Headache, abdominal pain, asthma, toothache and sore throat.

3.2.13.3 耳迷根
3.2.13.3 Root of Auricular Vagus Nerve

部位：在耳廓背与乳突交界处的耳根部。

Location: At the junction of retroauricle and mastoid, level with helix crus.

主治：头痛，鼻塞，胆道蛔虫症。

Indications: Headache, nasal obstruction and ascariasis of bile duct.

3.2.13.4 降压沟
3.2.13.4 Groove for Lowering Blood Pressure

部位：在耳廓背面，由内上方斜向外下方行走的凹沟处。

Location: Through the backside of superior antihelix crus and inferior antihelix crus, in the depression as a "Y" form.

主治：高血压。

Indications: Hypertension.

第四章 眼针疗法
CHAPTER FOUR EYE ACUPUNCTURE

眼针疗法是结合"观眼识病",根据病变部位,依中医脏腑经络学说,按八卦划分眼区,用毫针在眼眶周围相应的区域进行针刺,以治疗全身疾病的一种新的针刺疗法。

Eye acupuncture is a newly developed acupuncture method based on the theories "diagnosing deseases by observing the eye" as described in classical Chinese medical treaties. This method is useful for treatment of a wide variety of diseases. It utilizes needle stimulation of corresponding eye acupuncture points, distributed according to the Bagua (Eight Trigrams as specified in the *I Cjing*, Book of Changes).

4.1 眼针治疗的原理
4.1 The Principle of Eye Acupuncture

中医认为眼为精明之府,眼的功能活动与五脏六腑经络气血有着密切的联系。心主神明,目为心之使;肝开窍于目;五脏六腑之精气皆禀受于脾,上禀于目;肺主气,气帅血行目始得养;肾主水,肾旺水方化为津液,才能"尽上渗于目"。故《灵枢.大感论》指出"五脏六腑之精气,皆上注于目而为之精",又说"目者五脏六腑之精也,营卫魂魄之所常营也,神气之所生也"。说明目是五脏六腑精气

51

之所注,是人体营卫气血津液精神魂魄之所藏,而精气则是由经脉转输于目。人体经脉中足三阳均起于眼或其附近,而手三阳经皆有支脉止于眼或其附近,足厥阴肝经与手少阴心经与目系相通;奇经八脉中有阴跷脉、阳跷脉、任督脉与眼相连,而不与眼直接有关的经脉则通过表里联系,也间接与眼有关。所以《灵枢·邪气脏腑病形篇》言"十二经脉三百六十五络,其血气皆上于面而走空窍,其精阳气上于目而为精",《素问·五脏生成篇》有"诸脉者,皆属于目",《灵枢·口问》有"目者,宗脉之所聚也"的论述。

The eye is considered the "house of essence" in classic Chinese writings and its functional activities are very closely related to the Qi, Blood, Zang-fu organs, Channels and collaterals. Specifically, the heart controls the mental activities, and the eye is considered to be the window of the Heart. The Liver opens into the eyes. All the essence and energy transformed from the spleen ascends to the eye. The lungs govern Qi and only when Qi properly leads the circulation of the Blood can the eye be well "nourished." The Kidney governs water, and only the kidney is in full function can the water be turned into Jinye, which in turn irrigates the eyes. Hence, *Lingshu*: *Dahuo Lun* points out that "all the essence and energy of the five Zang-organs and six Fu-organs ascend to the eye and forms its "vision." It continues, "⋯ the eye is made from the essence of the five Zang-organs and six Fu-organs, it is the house of energy and mind, and it is the product of the vital energy." All this implies that the eye is a collection of essence and energy from all the internal organs; it is the bank of Yin energy, Wei energy, Qi, Blood, Jinye, and the mind. Meanwhile, it is the channels and collaterals that transmit essence and energy. Among the channels of the human body, all three FootYang channels originate at the eye or its vicinity; the three Hand—Yang channels have branches that terminate at the eye or its vicinity;

both the Foot—Jueyin Liver channel and the Hand—Shaoyin Heart channel communicate with the eye system; the Yinqiao, Yangqiao, Du. Ren channels of the eight extra channels group are connected to the eye. All the other channels not directly connected to the eye are indirectly related to the eye by way of the Exterior—Interior relationship. The *Lingshu: Xieqi Zangfu Bingxing Pain* explains that "···the Qi and Blood of all the 12 channels and 365 collaterals ascend to the face and enter the orifices, the pure and light part of the Qi and Blood enters the eye and forms ist vision." *Suwen: Wuzang Shengcheng Pain* says "···all the channels belong to the eye." *Lingshu Kouwen* says "···the eye is the collecting point of the converging channels."

由于目与脏腑关系密切,而且为五脏六腑之侯,故《灵枢·邪客》指出"因视目之五色,以知五脏而决死生,视其血脉,察其色,以知其寒热痛痹",《灵枢·四时气》认为"视其目色,以知病之存亡也"。《灵枢·论病诊尺》又指出"诊目病,赤脉从上下者,太阳病;从下上者,阳明病;从外走内者,少阳病","诊血脉者,多赤多热,多青多痛,多黑为久痹,多赤多黑多青皆见者,寒热"。

Since the eye is closely related to the Zang-Fu organs and is the window of the five Zang-organs and six FU-organs, *Lingshu, Xieke* points out "···by inspecting the five zangs and judge whether the patient will die or not; by inspecting the blood vessels of the eye and their colors, you can know whether the disease is of a Cold nature or Heat nature. and whether it involves pain or not." *Lingshu, Si Shi Qi* says that "···whether the disease is present or not can be deduced from the colors of the eye." *Lingshu Lunbin Zhenchi* again points out "···if the eye has red blood vessels going from superior to inferior, then the patient has Taiyang disease; if the blood vessels go from inferior to superior, the disease is of Yangming origin; if from lateral to medial, Shaoyang disease."and also,"…if the blood vessels are of a red color, the disease is of heat nature; green, pain; black, prolonged pain-syndrome; both red and black, chills and fever."

由此可见目不但与脏腑气血经络有着不可分割的联系,而且通过察目可识病,知病之所在,证之寒热虚实及其疾病的预后。因此,可以说眼针疗法是基于《内经》"观眼识病"的理论发展而来的。

Hence, it is obvious that the eye is very closely related to the Qi, Blood, channels and Zang-Fu organs. By inspecting the eye, one can diagnose diseases, locate them, and judge their nature—Cold, Heat, Excessive or Deficient—and discern the prognosis of the disease. Therefore, we can say that eye aacupuncture is a discipline that developed from the throries of Neijing for"diagnosing diseases by inspecting the eye."

4.2 眼针穴位分布及功效主治
4.2 The Locations Functions and Indications of the Eye Acupoints

眼针穴位分为"八区十三穴(如图 4—1)。

Eye acupoints are located in eight distinct areas around each eye and total 13 in number(see figure).

眼针穴位分布在距眼眶缘外 0.5cm 处,其中每个脏腑相应眼穴占 22.5°,而上、中、下焦各占 45°。

The eye acupoints are located 0.5 cm distal to the edge of the eye orbit. Each Zang—organ or Fu-organ point occupies an angle of 22.5 degrees while each area representing the Upper, Middle and Lower Warmers occupies an angle of 45 degrees.

各区所代表的脏腑可以治疗相应的脏腑或经络的病变。如心区能治疗心血管疾病及心经病。

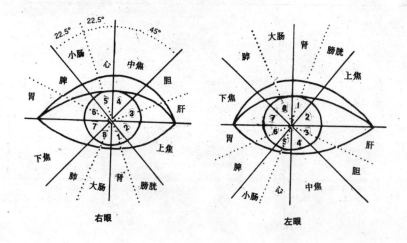

图 4.1　眼针穴位分布图

Each eye acupoint represents an organ and can be used to treat the Zang and Fu—organs or their related channels and their corresponding diseases. For example, the Heart eye acupoint may be needled to treat the diseases of both the cardiovascular system and the Heart channel.

上焦穴区主治膈肌以上疾病,包括头面、五官、上肢、胸背及心脏、肺脏、食管、气管等疾病。

The upper warmer eye acupoint is primarily used to treat diseases above the diaphragm including the head, the five sense organs, upper limbs, back and chest, heart, lungs, esophagus, trachea, etc.

中焦穴区主治膈以下、脐水平以上的疾病,包括腰背部和上腹部及所属区的内脏等疾病。

The Middle warmer eye acupoint is mainly used to treat the diseases between the levels of the diaphragm and the umbilicus, including the lumbar back region, epigastrium and the internal organs within this area.

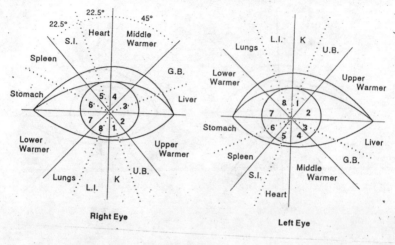

Fig 4.1 The Location of Eye Acupoints

下焦穴区主治脐水平以下疾病,包括腰骶部、盆腔、臀部、泌尿生殖系统及下肢等疾病.

the Lower Warmer eye acupoint is mainly used to treat the diseases below the level of the umbilicus, including the lumbosacral region, pelvic cavity, buttocks, urogenital system, and the lower limbs.

心包虽在形态上与心有别,但功能上却和心紧密联系,所以眼针穴位无心包。心包经病证可以针心穴。

The precardium is different from the Heart anatomically, but is closely related to it and has similar functions. Hence, there is no specific eye acupoint for the Pericardium, however, diseases of the Pericardium channel can be treated by needling the Heart eye acupoint.

4.3 眼针取穴原则
4.3 Method of Selecting Eye Acupoints

眼针取穴原则是以脏腑经络学说为指导,分为下列五种:
Selection is based on the classical Chinese medical theories regarding Zang—Fu organ systems and the channel system. There are five methods:

循经取穴:是根据中医经络辨证,依疾病症状属何经,即选相应经穴区。如咳嗽气喘、胸闷烦心,上臂前臂内侧前缘疼痛,属肺经病,即取肺穴区。

Corresponding—channel point selection: This is based on channel differentiation in which the point is selected on the corresponding disease—involved channel. For example, cough, asthma, fullness of the chest, fidgeting, and pain in the anterior—medial aspect of the upper limbs are all symptoms of the Lung channel imbalance, therefore, the eye acupoint Lung would be selected.

脏腑辨证取穴:根据中医脏腑辨证,证属何脏何腑,选取相应脏腑穴区。如眩晕属肝阳上亢者,取肝区;属肾虚者,取肾区;属脾虚痰浊中阻者取脾区。

Point selection according to Zang—Fu organs syndrome differentiation: For example, for vertigo, if caused by phlegm stagnation in the Middle warmer involving Spleen Deficiency, choose the eye acupoint Spleen; if it is caused by the hyperactivity of Liver Yang, choose the eye acupoint Liver; if it is caused by Kidney Deficiency, choose the eye acupoint kidney.

三焦取穴:根据三焦分布的部位对症取穴。如头面之疾寻上焦,腰骶及下肢之疾取下焦,脾胃之患取中焦。

Triple Warmer (San Jiao) point selection: According to the distribution of the Three Warmers, choose the corresponding Warmer point. For example, choose the eye acupoint Upper Warmer for diseases of the head and face; Middle warmer for diseases of the Spleen and Stomach; Lower Warmer for diseases of the lumbosacral region and lower limbs.

探穴法: 用三棱针柄在眼眶周穴区,用均衡力按压,出现酸麻胀重或发热发凉或不舒服感,是找到穴位的现象,可在反应点进行针刺。

Point—Detecting method: Using the end of the handle of a three—edged acupuncture needle, press along the eye acupoint area with an "even force." If the patient feels soreness, numbness, tenderness, heaviness or a cold, warm or an uncomfortable sensation being caused by needle pressure, then you have located an "indicated" piont. Needle this sensitive point.

观眼取穴: 是看白睛上血管形状及颜色的改变,不管什么病,只要在眼球区有明显的血管变化,即针该相应穴区.

Eye — Inspecting piont selection: When inspecting the changes in shape and coloration of the blood vessels in the whites of the eye, if an obvious change is observed, needle the corresponding eye acupoint.

4.4 眼针配穴原则举例

4.4 Examples of Eye Acupoint Treatment Prescriptions

中风偏瘫: 主穴:上焦区、下焦区。
配穴:伴高血压者加肝区,体虚加胃区,失语加心区。
Post—stroke hemiplegia: Main acupoints: upper and lower warmer;

Supplementary points: Liver, if hypertensive; Stomach, if weak; Heart, if has aphasia.

坐骨神经痛:主穴:下焦区。

配穴:足太阳型加膀胱区,足少阳型加胆区。

Sciatica: Main point: lower warmer; Sumpplementry points: UB if Foot Taiyang type; GB if Foot Shaoyang type.

肩周炎:主穴:上焦区。

配穴:大小肠区、心区。

Periarthritis of shoulder: Main point, upper warmer; Supplementary point, LI, SI and Heart.

头痛:主穴:上焦区。

配穴:前额头痛配大肠区、胃区,后头痛配膀胱区、小肠区,侧头痛配胆区,巅顶头痛配肝区。

Headache: Main point, upper warmer; Supplementary point, LI and Stomach if pain in forehead; GB, if pain in the lateral area; Liver, if pain in the top of the head.

胃脘痛:主穴:胃区,中焦区。

配穴:肝气犯胃型加肝区,脾虚者加脾区。

Stomachache: Main point: Middle warmer; Supplementary points: Liver, if caused by liver Qi invading stomach; Spleen, if Spleen deficiency.

呃逆:主穴:上焦区。

配穴:胃中寒加胃区,肝胃不和加肝、胃区。

Hiccup: Main point, Upper warmer, Supplementary points: Stomach, if caused by Cold in the stomach; Liver, if caused by disharmony of liver and stomach.

失眠:主穴:心区。

配穴:肝郁加肝区,心脾两虚加脾区,心肾不交加肾区。

Insomnia: Main point, Heart; Supplementary points: Liver if depression; Spleen, if deficiency of both Spleen and Heart; Kidney, if disharmony between kidney and heart.

胆绞痛：主穴：胆区、中焦区。

配穴：肝区。

Gall stone colic: Main point: GB and Middle warmer; Supplementary points, Liver.

腰痛：主穴：下焦区、膀胱区。

配穴：肾虚者加肾区，瘀血腰痛加肝区。

Lumbago: Main point: UB and Lower Warmer; if Kidney — deficiency, supplemented by Kidney; plus Liver point, if pain due to blood stasis.

痛经：主穴：下焦、肝区。

配穴：体虚加肾区、脾区。

Dysmenorrhea: Main Point: Lower Warmer and Liver; plus Kidney spleen, if week.

高血压：主穴：肝区。

配穴：肾虚加肾区，痰浊中阻加脾区。

Hypertension: Main point: Liver; plus Kidney, if Kidney — deficiency; plus Spleen if differentiated as phlegm accumlation.

心绞痛：心区、上焦区。

Angina Petrols: Main point: Heart and Upper warmer.

落枕：主穴：上焦。

配穴：不可以顾配小肠区，不可以俯仰取膀胱区。

Torticollis: Main point: Upper Warmer; if impairment of bowing head plus SI area; if impairment of lifting head, plus UB area.

4.5 眼针操作方法
4.5 The Manipulation of Eye Acupuncture

选好眼穴区,上眶是眉下际,下眶是离眼眶 0.5 cm 处,用 32号 0.5 寸或 1 寸不锈钢针。先以左手拇或食指压住眼球,并使眼眶皮肤绷紧,右手持针轻轻刺入,有针刺反应点的,可以直刺到 1—2分,按经区的可沿皮横刺 2—4 分,但不可超越所刺经区,直刺时达到骨膜即可,以有针感为度,留针 5—30 分钟。出针时用棉球压按针孔 2 分钟以防出血。

Choose the correct eye acupoint. Use a NO. 32, 0.5 inch or 1.0 inch long stainless steel needle. Press and fix the eyeball with the left thumb or the left index finger and tense the eyelid. Measwhile, gently insert the needle with the right hand.

When needling an "indicated" point, the needle can be inserted 0.1 —0.2 inch in depth strightly. If needling a given region, the needle can be inserted horizontally (transversely) at a depth of 0.2—0.4 cm, but not penetrating into another eye acupoint region.

When inserting strightly, the tip of needle may reach the membrance of bone. Make certain to obtain the needle sensation, then retain the needle for 5—30 minutes. Afterward, press the point(s) with cotton ball for more than 2 minutes to stop any bleeding.

第五章 子午流注针法
CHAPTER FIVE
ZIWU LIUZHU ACUPUNCTURE

5.1 天干地支的内容
5.1 Heavenly Stems and Earthly Branches

天干:甲、乙、丙、丁、戊、己、庚、辛、壬、癸。

Heavenly Stems(S):Jia(S1),Yi(S2),Bing(S3),Ding(S4),Wu(S5),Ji(S6),Geng(S7),Xin(S8),Ren(S9),Gui(S10).

地支:子、丑、寅、卯、辰、巳、午、未、申、酉、戌、亥。

Earthly Branches(B):Zi(B1),Chou(B2),Yin(B3),Mao(B4),Chen(B5),Si(B6),Wu(B7),Wei(B8),Shen(B9),You(B10),Xu(B11),Hai(B12).

5.2 子午流注针法的组成
5.2 The Constitution of Ziwu Liuzhu Acupuncture

5.2.1 天干配五行
5.2.1 Math 10 Heavenly Stems with Five Elements

天干	甲乙	丙丁	戊己	庚辛	壬癸
五行	木	火	土	金	水

Stems	S1 S2	S3 S4	S5 S6	S7 S8	S9 S10
Five Elements	Wood	Fire	Earth	Metal	Water

5.2.2 地支配五行
5.2.2 Match the 12 Earthly Branches With Five Elements

月份	一月	二月	三月	四月	五月	六月	七月	八月	九月	十月	十一月	十二月
地支	寅	卯	辰	巳	午	未	申	酉	戌	亥	子	丑
五行	木		土	火		土	金		土	水		土

Month	Jan.	Feb.	Mar.	Apr.	May	Jun.	Jul.	Aug.	Sep.	Oct.	Nov.	Dec.
B	B3	B4	B5	B6	B7	B8	B9	B10	B11	B12	B1	B2
Five Elements	Wood		Earth	Fire		Earth	Metal		Earth	Water		Earth

5.2.3 天干地支分配阴阳
5.2.3 Match the S and B with Yin and Yang

天干地支分配阴阳

阳天干	甲	丙	戊	庚	壬
阴天干	乙	丁	己	辛	癸

Yang   S1   S3   S5   S7   S9
Yin   S2   S4   S6   S8   S10

地支与阴阳相配

阳地支	子	寅	辰	午	申	戌
阴地支	丑	卯	巳	未	酉	亥

Yang   B1   B3   B5   B7   B9   B11
Yin   B2   B4   B6   B8   B10   B12

5.2.4 干支相配合成六十环周
5.2.4 Match the Stems and Branches to Form a Cycle of Sixty

干支相配合成六十环周是天干地支纪年、纪月、纪日、纪时的必用符号,列表如下:

Such a match is the fundation of the calculation of the year, the month, the day, and the times in Ziwu Liuzhu acupuncture.

干支配合六十环周表

甲子	乙丑	丙寅	丁卯	戊辰	己巳	庚午	辛未	壬申	癸酉
1	2	3	4	5	6	7	8	9	10
甲戌	乙亥	丙子	丁丑	戊寅	己卯	庚辰	辛巳	壬午	癸未
11	12	13	14	15	16	17	18	19	20
甲申	乙酉	丙戌	丁亥	戊子	己丑	庚寅	辛卯	壬辰	癸巳
21	22	23	24	25	26	27	28	29	30
甲午	乙未	丙申	丁酉	戊戌	己亥	庚子	辛丑	壬寅	癸卯
31	32	33	34	35	36	37	38	39	40
甲辰	乙巳	丙午	丁未	戊申	己酉	庚戌	辛亥	壬子	癸丑
41	42	43	44	45	46	47	48	49	50
甲寅	乙卯	丙辰	丁巳	戊午	己未	庚申	辛酉	壬戌	癸亥
51	52	45	54	55	56	57	58	59	60

Table Matching Stems With Branches of Form a Cycle of Sixty

1 S1B1	2 S2B2	3 S3B3	4 S4B4	5 S5B5	6 S6B6	7 S7B7	8 S8B8	9 S9B9	10 S10B10
11 S1B11	12 S2B12	13 S3B1	14 S4B2	15 S5B3	16 S6B4	17 S7B5	18 S8B6	19 S9B7	20 S10B8
21 S1B9	22 S2B10	23 S3B11	24 S4B12	25 S5B1	26 S6B2	27 S7B3	28 S8B4	29 S9B5	30 S10B6
31 S1B7	32 S2B8	33 S3B9	34 S4B10	35 S5B11	36 S6B12	37 S7B1	38 S8B2	39 S9B3	40 S10B4
41 S1B5	42 S2B6	43 S3B7	44 S4B8	45 S5B9	46 S6B10	47 S7B11	48 S8B12	49 S9B1	50 S10B2
51 S1B3	52 S2B4	53 S3B5	54 S4B6	55 S5B7	56 S6B8	57 S7B9	58 S8B10	59 S9B11	60 S10B12

5.2.5 一天十二时辰与 24 小时的分配
5.2.5 Twelve Branches match with the 24 hours in a day

时辰：	子	丑	寅	卯	辰	巳	午	未	申	酉	戌	亥
时间：	23-1	1-3	3-5	5-7	7-9	9-11	11-13	13-15	15-17	17-19	19-21	21-23
Branche	B1	B2	B3	B4	B5	B6	B7	B8	B9	B10	B11	B12
Time	23-1	1-3	3-5	5-7	7-9	9-11	11-13	13-15	15-17	17-19	19-21	21-23

5.2.6 年、月、日、时的干支推算法
5.2.6 The Calculation in Ziwu Liuzhu Acupuncture

5.2.6.1 年干支推算
5.2.6.1 The method of finding out the SB of the year

可依据"干支配合六十环周表"按顺序推出。如公元一九八四年为甲子年,则一九八五年为乙丑年,其余仿此。

From the table "Matching the Stems with Branches to Form a Cyle of 60" one may easily find out the SB of the year.

5.2.6.2 月干支推算法
5.2.6.2 Find out the SB of the month

每月的干支推算是按照农历计算的。为了应用方便,列表如下：

The monthe here is in lunar calendar. For the convenience of application, we may consult the following table.

月干支推算表

年份	月份（农历）											
	一月	二月	三月	四月	五月	六月	七月	八月	九月	十月	十一月	十二月
甲	丙寅	丁卯	戊辰	己巳	庚午	辛未	壬申	癸酉	甲戌	乙亥	丙子	丁丑
乙	戊寅	己卯	庚辰	辛巳	壬午	癸未	甲申	乙酉	丙戌	丁亥	戊子	己丑
丙	庚寅	辛卯	壬辰	癸巳	甲午	乙未	丙申	丁酉	戊戌	己亥	庚子	辛丑
丁	壬寅	癸卯	甲辰	乙巳	丙午	丁未	戊申	己酉	庚戌	辛亥	壬子	癸丑
戊	甲寅	乙卯	丙辰	丁巳	戊午	己未	庚申	辛酉	壬戌	癸亥	甲子	乙丑
己	丙寅	丁卯	戊辰	己巳	庚午	辛未	壬申	癸酉	甲戌	乙亥	丙子	丁丑
庚	戊寅	己卯	庚辰	辛巳	壬午	癸未	甲申	乙酉	丙戌	丁亥	戊子	己丑
辛	庚寅	辛卯	壬辰	癸巳	甲午	乙未	丙申	丁酉	戊戌	己亥	庚子	辛丑
壬	壬寅	癸卯	甲辰	乙巳	丙午	丁未	戊申	己酉	庚戌	辛亥	壬子	癸丑
癸	甲寅	乙卯	丙辰	丁巳	戊午	己未	庚申	辛酉	壬戌	癸亥	甲子	乙丑

Table Table for Finding Out the SB of the Month

Year	\ Month 1st	2nd	3rd	4th	5th	6th	7th	8th	9th	10th	11th	12th
S1	S3B3	S4B4	S5B5	S6B6	S7B7	S8B8	S9B9	S10B10	S1B11	S2B12	S3B1	S4B2
S2	S5B3	S6B4	S7B5	S8B6	S9B7	S10B8	S1B9	S2B10	S3B11	S4B12	S5B1	S6B2
S3	S7B3	S8B4	S9B5	S10B6	S1B7	S2B8	S3B9	S4B10	S5B11	S6B12	S7B1	S8B2
S4	S9B3	S10B4	S1B5	S2B6	S3B7	S4B8	S5B9	S6B10	S7B11	S8B12	S9B1	S10B2
S5	S1B3	S2B4	S3B5	S4B6	S5B7	S6B8	S7B9	S8B10	S9B11	S10B12	S1B1	S2B2
S6	S3B3	S4B4	S5B5	S6B6	S7B7	S8B8	S9B9	S10B10	S1B11	S2B12	S3B1	S4B2
S7	S5B3	S6B4	S7B5	S8B6	S9B7	S10B8	S1B9	S2B10	S3B11	S4B12	S5B1	S6B2
S8	S7B3	S8B4	S9B5	S10B6	S1B7	S2B8	S3B9	S4B10	S5B11	S6B12	S7B1	S8B2
S9	S9B3	S10B4	S1B5	S2B6	S3B7	S4B8	S5B9	S6B10	S7B11	S8B12	S9B1	S10B2
S10	S1B3	S2B4	S3B5	S4B6	S5B7	S6B8	S7B9	S8B10	S9B11	S10B12	S1B1	S2B2

5.2.6.3 日干支的推算

5.2.6.3 Calculation of SB of the day

由于农历的变化复杂,日干支的推算是按阳历进行的。计算时应先知道:①当年元旦干支的代数;②每月干支应加或应减数;③当天的日数。

Since the changes in lunar calendar is very complicated, so here we adopt the solar calendar. For the calculation, we must know (1). The SB of New Years Day (NYD) of a given year. (2). The constant number of SB of a given month. (3). The date of the given day.

公元 1992～2039 年元旦干支表

闰年		平年					
年份	元旦干支	年份	元旦干支	年份	元旦干支	年份	元旦干支
1992	丙子	1993	壬午	1994	丁亥	1995	壬辰
1996	丁酉	1997	癸卯	1998	戊申	1999	癸丑
2000	戊午	2001	甲子	2002	己巳	2003	甲戌
2004	己卯	2005	乙酉	2006	庚寅	2007	乙未
2008	庚子	2009	丙午	2010	辛亥	2011	丙辰
2012	辛酉	2013	丁卯	2014	壬申	2015	丁丑
2016	壬午	2017	戊子	2018	癸巳	2019	戊戌
2020	癸卯	2021	己酉	2022	甲寅	2023	己未
2024	甲子	2025	庚午	2026	乙亥	2027	庚辰
2028	丙戌	2029	辛卯	2030	丙申	2031	辛丑
2032	丁未	2033	壬子	2034	丁巳	2035	壬戌
2036	丁卯	2037	癸酉	2038	戊寅	2039	癸未

Table of the SB of New Years Day

Leap year		Common year					
Year	SB of NYD	Year	SB of NYD	Year		Year	SB of NYD
1992	S3B1	1993	S9B7	1994	S4B12	1995	S9B5
1996	S4B10	1997	S10B4	1998	S5B9	1999	S10B2
2000	S5B7	2001	S1B1	2002	S6B6	2003	S1B11
2004	S6B4	2005	S2B10	2006	S7B3	2007	S2B8
2008	S7B1	2009	S3B7	2010	S8B12	2011	S3B5
2012	S8B10	2013	S4B4	2014	S9B9	2015	S4B2
2016	S9B7	2017	S5B1	2018	S10B6	2019	S5B11
2020	S10B4	2021	S6B10	2022	S1B3	2023	S6B8
2024	S1B1	2025	S7B7	2026	S2B12	2027	S7B5
2028	S3B11	2029	S8B4	2030	S3B9	2031	S8B2
2032	S4B8	2033	S9B1	2034	S4B6	2035	S9B11
2036	S4B4	2037	S10B10	2038	S5B3	2039	S10B8

各月天干地支常数加减表

月份 \ 年别干支加减	平年 天干	平年 地支	闰年 天干	闰年 地支
一月	减一	减一	减一	减一
二月	加零	加六	加零	加六
三月	减二	加十		
四月	减一	加五		
五月	减一	减一		
六月	加零	加六	余数加一	
七月	加零	加零		
八月	加一	加七		
九月	加二	加二		
十月	加二	加八		
十一月	加三	加三		
十二月	加三	加九		

Table of Constant Number of Monthly SB

Month	common year		leap year	
	S	B	S	B
1st	−1	−1	−1	−1
2nd	0	6	0	6
3rd	−2	10		
4th	−1	5		
5th	−1	−1		
6th	0	6		
7th	0	0	Remainder+1	
8th	1	7		
9th	2	2		
10th	2	8		
11th	3	3		
12th	3	9		

了解到上述三项数目之后,即可按下述两个公式推算日干支。

天干计算公式:

(当年元旦天干代数+所求日数+当月天干加减常数)÷10=商……余数(余数就是天干代表数。如果余数为0,则为癸日)。

地支计算公式:

(当年元旦地支代数+所求日数+当月地支加减常数)÷12=商……余数(余数即为地支代数。如果余数为0,则为亥日)。

闰年3月之后各月天干地支常数余数加1。

The formula for the calculation of SB of a given day:

(The substitution number of S of the NYD + the constant number of S of the given month + Date of the month)/10 = Quotient……Remainder (acquired substitution number of S; if the remainder is zero, then the S of that day will be S10).

(The substitution number of B of the NYD + the constant number of B of the given month + Date of that month)/12 = Quotient……Remainder (acquired substitution number of B; if the remainder is zero, then the B of that day will be B12).

In a leap year, we should add one to the substitution number of SB from March, since there is one more day in February.

5.2.6.4 时干支的推算
5.2.6.4 Find out the SB of the Time Division of a day (TD)

各日时辰干支表

干支\时辰\日	子时	丑时	寅时	卯时	辰时	巳时	午时	未时	申时	酉时	戌时	亥时
甲日、己日	甲子	乙丑	丙寅	丁卯	戊辰	己巳	庚午	辛未	壬申	癸酉	甲戌	乙亥
乙日、庚日	丙子	丁丑	戊寅	己卯	庚辰	辛巳	壬午	癸未	甲申	乙酉	丙戌	丁亥
丙日、辛日	戊子	己丑	庚寅	辛卯	壬辰	癸巳	甲午	乙未	丙申	丁酉	戊戌	己亥
丁日、壬日	庚子	辛丑	壬寅	癸卯	甲辰	乙巳	丙午	丁未	戊申	己酉	庚戌	辛亥
戊日、癸日	壬子	癸丑	甲寅	乙卯	丙辰	丁巳	戊午	己未	庚申	辛酉	壬戌	癸亥

Table for Finding Out Td SB in a Day

Day \ Td	B1	B2	B3	B4	B5	B6	B7	B8	B9	B10	B11	B12
S1,S6	S1B1	S2B2	S3B3	S4B4	S5B5	S6B6	S7B7	S8B8	S9B9	S10B10	S1B11	S2B12
S2,S7	S3B1	S4B2	S5B3	S6B4	S7B5	S8B6	S9B7	S10B8	S1B9	S2B10	S3B11	S4B12
S3,S8	S5B1	S6B2	S7B3	S8B4	S9B5	S10B6	S1B7	S2B8	S3B9	S4B10	S5B11	S6B12
S4,S9	S7B1	S8B2	S9B3	S10B4	S1B5	S2B6	S3B7	S4B8	S5B9	S6B10	S7B11	S8B12
S5,S10	S9B1	S10B2	S1B3	S2B4	S3B5	S4B6	S5B7	S6B8	S7B9	S8B10	S9B11	S10B12

5.2.7 天干地支与脏腑经络相配
5.2.7 Match the S and B with Zang—fu organs and Meridians

天干与经络脏腑相配表

十天干	甲	乙	丙	丁	戊	己	庚	辛	壬	癸
脏腑经络	胆	肝	小肠 三焦	心 心包	胃	脾	大肠	肺	膀胱	肾

The ten Heavenly Stems and Zang-Fu Organs (Meridian)

Stems	S1	S2	S3	S4	S5	S6	S7	S8	S9	S10
Organs and Meridians	GB	LR	SI SJ	HT PC	ST	SP	LI	LU	UB	KI

地支与脏腑经络相配表

地支	寅	卯	辰	巳	午	未	申	酉	戌	亥	子	丑
脏腑经络	肺	大肠	胃	脾	心	小肠	膀胱	肾	心包	三焦	胆	肝

Earthly Branches and Zang—Fu Organs(Meridian)

Branches	B3	B4	B5	B6	B7	B8	B9	B10	B11	B12	B1	B2
Organs and maidians	LU	LI	ST	SP	HT	SI	BL	KI	PC	SJ	GB	LR

5.3 子午流注纳子法
5.3 The Method of Adopting Branches

5.3.1 纳子法的含义
5.3.1 The implication of adopting branches

"纳子法"是以一天十二时辰配合十二经脉(见"地支配合脏腑经络表)按时开穴。

This method is to match the 12 time division in a day with the corresponding Zang—Fu organs and meridians, and to select corresponding points in relevant time division.

5.3.2 补母泻子取穴法

5.3.2 Select points according to the principle of invigorating the "Mother" and reducing the "Child"

这也是根据脏腑配合时辰,结合各经症状的虚实,通过将十二经脉的五输穴配五行,按照"虚则补其母,实则泻其子"的原则取穴治疗。具体开穴见"子午流注纳子法补母泻子取穴表"。

Based on the match of Zang—Fu organs and time division, and on the match of five elements and five—shu points in 12 channels; the points are selected according to the principle of invigorating the "Mother" and reducing "Child". (See table below)

子午流注纳子法补母泻子取穴表

经别	五行	流注时间	病症	补法 母穴	补法 时间	泻法 子穴	泻法 时间	本穴	原穴
肺	辛金	寅	咳喘、胸满、心烦	大渊	卯	尺泽	寅	经渠	太渊
大肠	庚金	卯	齿痛、咽喉鼻疾患	曲池	辰	二间	卯	商阳	合谷
胃	戊土	辰	腹胀、脚气	解溪	巳	厉兑	辰	足三里	冲阳
脾	己土	巳	黄疸、便溏	大都	午	商丘	巳	太白	太白
心	丁火	午	舌痛、心悸、失眠	少冲	未	神门	午	少府	神门
小肠	丙火	未	颈项痛、肩痛	后溪	申	小海	未	阳谷	腕骨
膀胱	壬水	申	头项痛、腰背痛	至阴	酉	束骨	申	通谷	京骨
肾	癸水	酉	心悸、腰痛	复溜	戌	涌泉	酉	阴谷	太溪
心包络	丁火	戌	心烦、肋痛	中冲	亥	大陵	戌	劳宫	大陵
三焦	丙火	亥	耳聋、眼痛	中渚	子	天井	亥	支沟	阳池
胆	甲木	子	头痛、肋痛	侠溪	丑	阳辅	子	足临泣	丘墟
肝	乙木	丑	疝气、肋痛	曲泉	寅	行间	丑	大敦	太冲

Table Selecting Points According to the Principle of Invigorating the "Mother" and Reducing the "Child"

Channels	Five Elements	Wax Td	Symptoms and Signs	Invigoration "Mother"	Td	Reduction "Child"	Td	Original Point	Source Point
LU	S8Metal	B3	Cough &dyspnea, fullness of the chest, vexation	LU_9	B_4	Lu_5	Lu_8	Lu_9	
LI	S7Metal	B4	Toothache, nasal & laryngoparyngeal diseases	LI_{11}	B5	LI_2	B4	LI_1	LI_4
ST	S5Earth	B5	Abdominal distention, beriberi	sT_{41}	B6	St_{45}	B5	ST_{36}	ST_{42}
SP	S6Earth	B6	Jaundice, loose bowel	Sp_2	B7	Sp_5	B6	Sp_3	Sp_3
HT	S4Fire	B7	Glossalgia, palpitation, insomnia	HT_9	B8	H_7	B7	H_8	H_7
SI	S3Fire	B8	Pain of the neck, nape, shoulder	SI_3	B9	SI_8	B8	SI_5	SI_4
BL	S9Water	B9	Pain of the head, nape, back, lumbago	Bl_{67}	B10	BL_{65}	B9	BL_{66}	BL_{64}
KI	S10Water	B10	Palpiation, lumbago	KI_7	B_{11}	KI_1	B10	KI_{10}	KI_3
Pc	S4Fire	B11	Vexation, hypochondriac pain	PC_9	B_{12}	PC_7	B11	PC_8	Pc_7
SJ	S3Fire	B12	Deafness, eye pain	SJ_3	B1	SJ_{10}	B12	SJ_6	SJ_4
GB	S1Wood	B1	Headache, hypochondriac pain	GB_{43}	B2	GB_{38}	B1	GB_{41}	GB_{40}
LR	S2Wood	B2	Hernia, hypochondriac pain	LR_{18}	B3	LR2	B2	LR1	LR_3

5.3.3 某时配某经

5.3.3 Ceratain time division match with certain chanb

该法根据时辰与脏腑经络相配的原理,在某一特定的时辰内,与该时辰相配经脉上的所有穴位均可选用。

In this method, every point in the Channel corrsponding to a given time division could be selected in this time division.

如:每日寅时,相应的经脉是肺经,此时肺经上从中府到少商的所有穴位均可选用来治疗肺及相关脏腑经络病变。

For example, every morning in B3 time division, Lung vital energy streams down along the arm, from LU1 to LU ll, all eleven points in Lung channel may be seleced to treat the disorders of Lung and relevant organs.

5.4 子午流注纳甲法
5.4 The Method of Adopting Stems

5.4.1 含义
5.4.1 Implication

此法是子午流注针法的主要部分。它用来诊时的日、时干支,结合人体经脉气血的流注及五行相生规律按顺序开穴。

This is the most important method of Ziwu Liuzhu acupuncture. The points are selected according to the time division when a patient calls on and ask for treatment. Also the law of the circulation of Qi and blood, and the rule of mutual generation between five elements are also taken into account.

5.4.2 纳甲法开穴原则
5.4.2 Principle of point selection

(1)阳日阳时开阳经;阴日阴时开阴经。即阳日开阳经井穴开始,按井、荥、输、经、合依次于阳时开穴,十二时辰开完则转注次日再开阳时。阴经阴时道理同此。

(1) At Yang time division on Yang day, select points of Yang meridians; at Yin time division of Yin day, select points from Yin meridians. Starting from Jing (well) point, then the others of five-shu points.

(2)返本归原。每当开到"输穴"时要同时开值日经原穴,阴经无原穴则以"输"代原穴。

(2) Select the Yuan (source) point of the On－duty meridian, while a Shu (stream) point is selected. Since there are no Yuan points in Yin meridians, they are substituted by Shu (stream) points in On－duty meridian. This princple is also called "return to the root and come back to the source".

(3)气纳三焦,开生我穴:三焦主持诸气,气为阳,所以凡是阳经开到合穴,下一阳经便应"气纳三焦,开生我穴"。这里"我"指的是值日阳经。如值日经是胆经,属木,木之母穴属水,所以当胆经值日到了壬午时辰开胆经合穴时,下一阳时甲申便要开三焦经属水的荥穴液门(水生木)。

Triple warmer receives Qi: select the "Mother" points in Triple Warmer meridian (Sanjiao Meridian)

Triple Warmer is regarde the "father" of the Yang Qi. Whenever a He (sea) point in a Yang meridian is selected, the "Mother" point (the element corresponding to this "mother" point generates the element corresponding to the On－duty Yang meridian) should be selected after.

For instance, if Gallbladder is on duty, since ito attribute is Wood, its "Mother" Point in Triple Warmer meridian belongs to Water. Therefore, Yimen (SJ 2) is used.

(4)血归包络,开我生穴:血归包络,血为阴;所以凡是阴经开到合穴时,下一阴经时辰就要血归包络,开(心包经)"我"生之穴。

这里"我"指值日阴经。比如肝经值日当开到癸巳时,选用肾经合穴阴谷,这样下一时辰乙未就要选劳营(心包经火穴,取木生火之意)

(4) Blood belongs to Pericardium; select the "Child" point in Pericardium meridian.

Blood possesses the property of Yin; all Yin blood converge to Pericardium. Whenever a He (sea) point in a Yin meridian is selected, the "Child" point (The element corresponding to the "Child" point is generated by the element attributed to the On—duty Yin meridian) should be selected next.

For an example, if Liver meridian is on—duty, since its attribute is Wood, its "Child" point in Pericardium meridian will attribute to Fire. Therefore the Laogong (PC 8) is used.

5.4.3 纳甲法逐日开穴表
5.4.3 Table for Point Selection in the Method of Adopting Stems

掌握了以上开穴原则,结合前面介绍的年、月、日、时的干支推算,便可推算出逐日所开的穴位。下列各表列出逐日开穴。

After mastering the above principles and based on the calculation of SB of year, month, day and time division, one may infer exact point at each given time division. As to details, the folloring tables list all points selection in adopting stems method.

甲(胆 主 气)日

时辰：甲戌——丙子——戊寅——庚辰——壬午——甲申
经脉：胆 — 小肠 — 胃 — 大肠 — 膀胱 — 三焦
穴性：井 — 荥 — 输 — 经 — 合 — 荥
　　　　　　　　　　　　│
穴位：窍阴——前谷——陷谷——阳溪——委中——液门
　　　　　　　　　　　　│
　　　　　　　　　　　丘墟

Stems S1 Day (Gallbladder channel on Duty)

Td	S1B11	S3B1	S5B3	S7B5	S9B7	S1B9
Channel	GB	SI	ST	LI	BL	SJ
Nature of Point	Well	Spring	Stream	River	Sea	Spring
	GB_{44}	SI_2	ST_{43}	LI_5	BV_{40}	SJ_2
			Needle GB_{40} simultaneously			

乙(肝 主 气)日

时辰：乙酉——丁亥——己丑——辛卯——癸巳——乙未
经脉：肝 — 心 — 脾 — 肺 — 肾 — 心包
穴性：井 — 荥 — 俞 — 经 — 合 — 荥
穴位：大敦——少府——太白——经渠——阴谷——劳宫
　　　　　　　　　　│
　　　　　　　　　太冲

S2 Day (Liver Channel on Duty)

Td	S2B10	S4B12	S6B2	S8B4	S10B8	S2B8
Channel	LR	HT	Sp	Lu	KI	Pc
Nature of Poitn	Well	Spring	Sream	River	Sea	Spring
	LR_1	HT_8	SP_3	LU_8	KI_{10}	PC_8
			Needle LR_3 simultaneosly			

丙(小肠主气)日

时辰：丙 申 —— 戊 戌 —— 庚 子 —— 壬 寅 —— 甲 辰 —— 丙 午
经脉：小 肠 —— 胃 —— 大 肠 —— 膀 胱 —— 胆 —— 三 焦
穴性：井 —— 荥 —— 俞 —— 经 —— 合 —— 俞
穴位：少 泽 —— 内 庭 —— 三 间 —— 昆 仑 —— 阳陵泉 —— 中 渚
　　　　　　　　　　　　　　|
　　　　　　　　　　　　　腕骨

S3 Day (Small Intestine channel on Duty)

Td	S3B9	S5B11	S7B1	S9B3	S1B5	S3B7
channel	SI	ST	LI	BL	GB	ST
Nature of Point	Well	Spring	Stream	River	Sea	Stream
	SI_1	ST_{44}	LI_3	BL_{60}	GB_{34}	ST_3
			Needle SI_4 Simultaneously			

丁(心　主　气)日

时辰：丁末——己酉——辛亥——癸丑——乙卯——丁巳
经脉：心　——　脾　——　肺　——　肾　——　肝　——　心包
穴性：井　——　荥　——　俞　——　经　——　合　——　俞
穴位：少冲——大都——太渊——复溜——曲泉——大陵
　　　　　　　　　　　　　｜
　　　　　　　　　　　　神门

Td	S4 Day (Heart Channel on Duty)					
	S4B8	S6B10	S8B12	S10B2	S2B4	S4B6
Channel	HT	SP	Lu	KI	LR	PC
Nature of Point	Well	Spring	Stream	River	Sea	Stream
	HT_9	SP_2	Lu_9	KI_7	LR_8	PC_7
	Needle HT_7 simultaneously.					

戊(胃　主　气)日

时辰：戊午——庚申——壬戌——甲子——丙寅——戊辰
经脉：胃　——大肠——膀胱——　胆　——小肠——三焦
穴性：井　——　荥　——　俞　——　经　——　合　——　经
穴位：厉兑——二间——束骨——阳辅——小海——支沟
　　　　　　　　　　　　　｜
　　　　　　　　　　　　冲阳

S5 Day (Stomach Channel on Duty)

Td	S5B7	S7B9	S9B11	S1B1	S3B3	S5B5
Channel	ST	LI	BL	GB	SI	SJ
Nature of Poin	Well ST_{45}	Spring LI_2	Stream BL_{65}	River GB_{38}	Sea SI_8	River SJ_6
			Needle ST_{42} simultaneously			

己（脾 主 气）日

时辰：己巳——辛未——癸酉——乙亥——丁丑——己卯
经脉：脾——肺——肾——肝——心——心包
穴性：井——荥——俞——经——合——经
穴位：隐白——鱼际——太溪——中封——少海——间使
　　　　　　　　　　　|
　　　　　　　　　　太白

S6 Day (Spleen Channel on Duty)

Td	S6B6	S8B8	S10B10	S2B12	S4B2	S6B4
Channel	SP	LU	KI	LR	HT	PC
Nature of Point	Well SP_1	Spring LU_{10}	Stream KI_3	River LR_4	Sea HT_3	River PC_5
			Needle Sp_3 simultaneously			

庚(大肠主气)日

时辰：庚 辰――壬 午――甲 申――丙 戌――戊 子――庚 寅
经脉：大 肠――膀 胱――胆――小 肠――胃――三 焦
穴性：井――荥――俞――经――合――合
穴位：商 阳――通 谷――足临泣――阳 谷――足三里――天 井
　　　　　　　　　　　　　|
　　　　　　　　　　　　合谷

S7 Day (Large Intestine Channel on Duty)

Td	S7B5	S9B7	S1B9	S3B11	S5B1	S7B3
Channel	LI	BL	GB	SI	ST	SJ
Nature of Point	Well LI_1	Spring BL_{66}	Stream GB_{41}	River SI_5	Sea ST_{36}	Sea ST_{10}
			Needle LI_4 simultaneously			

辛(肺主气)日

时辰：辛 卯――癸 巳――乙 未――丁 酉――己 亥――辛 丑
经脉：肺――肾――肝――心――脾――心包
穴性：井――荥――俞――经――合――合
穴位：少 商――然 谷――太 冲――灵 道――阴陵泉――曲 泽
　　　　　　　　　　　　　|
　　　　　　　　　　　　太渊

S8 Day (Lung Channel on Duty)

Td	S8B4	S10B6	S2B8	S4B10	S6B12	S8B2
Channel	LU	KI	LR	H	Sp	PC
Nature of Point	Well Lu_{11}	Spring KI_2	Stream LR_3	River H_4	Sea Sp_9	Sea PC_3
			Needle LU_9 simul taneously			

壬（膀胱主气）日

时辰：壬寅——甲辰——丙午——戊申——庚戌——壬子
经脉：膀胱——胆——小肠——胃——大肠——三焦
穴性：井——荥——俞——经——合——井
穴位：至阴——侠溪——后溪——解溪——曲池——关冲
　　　　　　　　　　　　　　　|
　　　　　京骨，阳池

S6 Day (Urinary Bladder Channel on Duty)

Td	S9B3	S1B5	S3B7	S5B9	S7B11	S9B1
Channel	BL	GB	SI	ST	LI	SJ
Nature of Point	Well BL_{67}	Spring GB_{43}	Stream SI_3	River ST_{41}	Sea LI_{11}	Well SJ_1
			Needle BL_{64}, SJ_4 simultaneously			

癸(肾 主 气)日

时辰： 癸亥——乙丑——丁卯——己巳——辛未——癸酉
经脉： 肾 —— 肝 —— 心 —— 脾 —— 肺 —— 心包
穴性： 井 —— 荥 —— 俞 —— 经 —— 合 —— 井
穴位： 涌泉——行间——神门——商丘——尺泽——中冲
　　　　　　　　　　　　　　　　　　　　|
　　　　　　　大陵,太溪

S10 Day (Kiney Channel on Duty)

Td	S10B12	S2B2	S4B4	S6B6	S8B8	S10B10
Channel	KI	LR	HT	SP	Lu	PC
Nature of Point	Well KI_1	Spring LR_2	Stream HT_7	River Sp_5	Sea Lu_5	Well PC_9
			Needle PC_7, KI_3 simultaneously			

下 篇
常见病的针灸治疗

PART TWO
THE TREATMENT OF COMMON DISEASES

第一章 内科病证
CHAPTER ONE INTERNAL DISEASES

1.1 中风
1.1 Wind Stroke

中风是一种急性疾病,它以突然昏仆、不省人事、半身不遂、言语不清或口㖞为主要表现。它起病急骤,变化迅速而似"风",故名中风。

Wind stroke is an emergency manifested by falling down in a fit with loss of consciousness, or hemiplegia, slurred speech and deviated mouth. It is characterized by abrupt onset with pathological changes varying quickly like the wind, from which the term "wind stroke" comes.

1.1.1 辨证
1.1.1 Differentiation

1.1.1.1 中脏腑
1.1.1.1 Attack on the zang—fu organs

闭证:
Tense syndrome:

主要表现：突然昏仆，神识昏昧，两手紧握，牙关紧闭，面赤气粗，喉中痰鸣，二便不通，脉弦滑有力。

Main manifestations: Falling down in a fit with loss of consciousness, tightly closed hands and clenched jaws, flushed face, coarse breathing, rattling in the throat, retention of urine, constipation, red tongue with thick yellow or dark grey coating, string—taut, rolling and forceful pulse.

脱证：

Flaccid syndrome:

主要表现：突然昏仆，神识昏昧，目合口张，鼻鼾息微，四肢软瘫，小便失禁，舌痿软，脉细弱。重者四肢逆冷，面红如妆，脉来浮大。

Main manifestations: Falling down in a fit and sudden loss of consciousness with mouth agape and eyes closed, snoring but feeble breathing, flaccid paralysis of limbs, incontinence of urine, flaccid tongue, thready, weak pulse, and in severe cases cold limbs, or flushing of face as rouged, fading or big floating pulse.

1.1.1.2 中经络

1.1.1.2 Attack on the meridians and collaterals

主要表现：半身不遂，肢体麻木，口角㖞斜，言语不清，伴见头痛，眩晕，肌肉抽掣，面目红赤，口渴咽干，烦躁，脉弦滑。

Main manifestations: Hemiplegia, numbness of the limbs, deviated mouth, slurring of speech, accompanied by headache, dizziness, vertigo, twitching of muscles, red eyes and flushed face, thirst, dryness of the throat, irritability, string-taut and rolling pulse.

1.1.2 治疗

1.1.2 Treatment

1.1.2.1 中脏腑

1.1.2.1 Attack on the zang—fu organs

闭证:

Tense syndrome:

百会、水沟、丰隆、太冲、涌泉、十二井穴。

牙关紧闭者加下关、合谷、颊车;舌强语謇加哑门、廉泉、通里。

Baihui(DU 20), Shuigon (DU 26), Fenglong(ST 40), Taichong (LR 3), Yongquan(KI 1), twelve Jing—(well) points on both hands (LU11,HT9,PC9,LI1,SJ1,SI1)

For clenched jaws, adding Xiaguan(ST7), Jiache(ST6), Hegu (LI4); and for aphasia and stiffness of tongue, Yamen(DU15), Lianquan(RN23), and Tongli(HT5).

脱证:

Flaccid syndrome:

施以灸法于任脉俞穴以回阳救逆。

处方:神阙(隔盐灸)、气海、关元。

Moxibustion is apppplied to points of the Ren meridian to restore yang from collapse.

Prescription: Shenque (RN8) indirect moxibustion with salt, Qihai(RN6), Guanyuan(RN4).

1.1.2.2 中经络

1.1.2.2 Attack on the meridians and collaterals.

主要选取阳经及督脉之穴位以熄风、调通气血。先针健侧,继针患侧。

处方:百会、通天、风府。

上肢:肩髃、曲池、外关、合谷;

下肢:环跳、阳陵泉、足三里、解溪;

口㖞:地仓、颊车。

Points along the DU meridian and the Yang meridians of the affected side are mainly used to regulate Qi and blood, remove obstruction from the meridians and collaterals and reduce the wind. Needling the healthy side first, then affected side.

Prescription: Baihui(DU20), Tongtian(BL7), Fengfu(DU16).
Upper limbs: Jianyu(LI15), Quchi(LI11), Waiguan(SJ5), Hegu(LI4).

Lower limbs: Huantiao(GB30), Yanglingquan(GB34), Zusanli(ST36), Jiexi(ST41).

Deviated mouth: Dicang(ST4), Jiache(ST6).

注:该症相当於现代医学之脑出血、脑栓塞、脑血栓形成、蛛网膜下腔出血等。

Remark: The wind stroke is referred to cerebral hemorrhage, thrombosis, embolism, subachnoid hemorrhage, etc. in modern medicine.

1.2 感 冒
1.2 Common Cold

1.2.1 辨证
1.2.1 Differentiation

1.2.1.1 风寒
1.2.1.1 Wind cold

主要表现:发热恶寒,无汗头痛,肢体酸痛,鼻塞流涕,咽痒咳嗽,声音嘶哑,痰多而稀,舌苔薄白,脉浮紧。

Main manifestations: Chills, fever, anhidrosis, headache, soreness and pain of the limbs, nasal obstruction, running nose, itching of the throat, cough, hoarse voice, profuse thin sputum, thin white tongue coating, superficial and tense pulse.

1.2.1.2 风热
1.2.1.2 Wind heat

主要表现：发热汗出,微微恶风,头胀痛,咳嗽黄粘痰,咽喉肿痛,口渴,薄白或薄黄苔,脉象浮数。

Main manifestation: Fever, sweating, slight aversion to wind, pain and distending sensation of the head, cough with yellow, thick sputum, congested and sore throat, thirst, thin white or yellowish tongue coating, superficial and rapid pulse.

1.2.2 治疗
1.2.2 Treatment

1.2.2.1 风寒
1.2.2.1 Wind cold

选督脉、太阳、少阳经穴,针以泻法以驱散风寒。体弱者施以平补平泻及灸法。

处方:风府、风门、风池、合谷。

Reducing method is used to the points of the Du, Taiyang and Shaoyang channels to eliminate wind cold and relieve exterior symptoms. Even method combined with moxibustion would be applied to patients with weak constitutions.

Prescription: Fengfu (DU16), Fengmen (BL12), Fengchi (GB20), Hegu (LI4).

1.2.2.2 风热

1.2.2.2 Wind heat

选取督脉、少阳、阳明经穴,针以泻法以疏散风热。

处方:大椎、曲池、外关、合谷、鱼际、少商。

Reducing method is applied to the points of the Du, Shaoyang and Yangming channels to eliminate wind heat evil.

Prescription: Dazhui(DU14), Quchi(LI11), Waiguan(SJ5), Hegu(LI 4),Yuji(LU10),Shaoshang (LU 11).

1.3 咳嗽
1.3 Cough

1.3.1 辨证
1.3.1 Differentiation

1.3.1.1 风寒型
1.3.1.1 Wind—cold type

主要表现:咳嗽,咽痒,痰白而稀,恶寒发热,头痛无汗,鼻塞流涕,舌苔薄白,脉浮。

Main manifestations: Cough, itching in the throat, thin and white sputum, aversion to cold, fever, anhidrosis, headache, nasal obstructuion and discharge, thin, white tongue coating and superficial pulse.

1.3.1.2 风热型
1.3.1.2 Wind—heat type;

主要表现:咳嗽痰黄稠,呛咳,口渴,咽痛,发热或头痛,恶风汗出,舌苔黄,脉浮数。

Main manifestations: Cough with yellow, thick sputum, choking cough, thirst, sore throat, fever, or headache, aversion to wind, sweating, thin, yellow tongue coating, superficial and rapid pulse.

1.3.1.3 痰湿阻肺
1.3.1.3 Blockage of the lung by phlegm;

主要表现：咳嗽痰多，痰白而粘，胸闷，纳呆，舌苔白腻，脉滑。

Main manifestations: Cough with profuse, white and sticky sputum, stuffiness and depression of the chest, loss of appetite, white, sticky tongue coating and rolling pulse.

1.3.1.4 肝火犯肺
1.3.1.4 Injury of the lung by Liver—fire

主要表现：咳嗽胁痛，气逆作咳，痰少而粘，面色红赤，咽干，舌苔黄干，脉弦数。

Main manifestations: Cough with the pain in hypochondriac region, cough often caused by adverse ascending of Qi, scanty and sticky sputum, flushed face, dry throat, yellow and dry coating of tongue, string—taut and rapid pulse.

1.3.1.5 阴虚肺燥
1.3.1.5 Dryness of the lung with deficiency of yin

主要表现：干咳，无痰或少痰，咽干鼻燥，喉痛，痰中有血丝或甚则咳血，午后潮热，面潮红，舌红少苔，脉细数。

Main manifestations: Dry cough without sputum or with scanty sputum, dryness of the nose and throat, sore throat, spitting blood or even coughing blood, afternoon fever, malar flush, red tongue, thin coating, thready and rapid pulse.

1.3.2 治疗
1.3.2 Treatmeant

1.3.2.1 风寒、风热型

1.3.2.1 Type of wind—cold and wind—heat

主要选取手太阴及手阳明经穴为主,风寒者针灸并施,风热者只针不灸。

处方:列缺、合谷、肺俞。

咽喉肿痛加少商,恶寒发热加大椎、外关。

The points from the Taiyin and Yangming channels of Hand are slected as the principal ones. In case of wind-cold type, both acupuncture and moxibustion would be applied, while in case of wind heat type only acupuncture is used.

Prescription: Lieque(LU 7), Hegu(LI 4), Feishu(BL 13); for pain and swelling of the throat, plus Shaoshang(LU 11); for fever and aversion to cold, Dazhui(DU 14) and Waiguan(SJ 5).

1.3.2.2 痰湿阻肺

1.3.2.2 Blocage of the lung by phlegm

处方:肺俞、中脘、尺泽、足三里、丰隆。

针时可补泻并用,或配以灸法。

Prescription: Feishu(BL 13), Zhongwan(RN 12), Chize(LU 5), Zusanli(ST 36), Fenglong(ST 40).

Both reinforcing and reducing methods should be considered in acupuncture treatment, or combined with moxibustion to strengthen the function of the spleen.

1.3.2.3 肝火犯肺

1.3.2.3 Injury of lung by liver-fire

处方:肺俞、尺泽、阳陵泉、太冲。

针足厥阴肝经穴以泻法,施以平补平泻法于手太阴肺经穴。不灸。

Prescription: Feishu(BL 13), Chize(LU 5), Yanglingquan(GB

34),Taichong(LR 3).

Needle the points of Liver channel of foot—Jueyin with reducing method; and needle the points of Lung channel with even method. No moxibustion.

1.3.2.4 阴虚肺燥
1.3.2.4 Deficiency of Yin with dryness of the lung

处方：肺俞、中府、列缺、照海。

施以平补平泻以肃肺润燥。

如果有咯血加孔最、膈俞。

Prescription: Feishu(BL 13), Zhongfu(LU 1), Lieque(LU 7), Zhaohai(KI 6)

Even method is applied in acupuncture to eliminate dryness and descend lung Qi.

In case of hemoptysis, plus Kongzui(LU 6)and Geshu(BL 17).

1.4 哮喘
1.4 Asthma

1.4.1 辨证
1.4.1 Differentiation

1.4.1.1 风寒型
1.4.1.1 Wind—cold type

主要表现：咳嗽痰稀，呼吸急促，喉中痰鸣，伴发热恶寒头痛，早期无汗，口不渴，舌苔白，脉浮紧。

Main manifestations: Cough with thin sputum, rapid breathing, accompanied by chills, fever, headache, and anhidrosis at the early stage, absence of thirst, white tongue coating, superficial and tense pulse.

1.4.1.2 痰热型
1.4.1.2 Phlegm—heat type

主要表现:呼吸急促而短,声高气粗,咳嗽痰黄粘,胸闷,发热烦躁,口干,舌苔黄腻,脉滑数。

Main manifestations: Rapid and short breathing, strong and coarase voice, cough with thick yellow sputum, sensation of chest stuffiness, fever, restlessness, dryness of the mouth, thick yellow or sticky coating, rolling and rapid pulse.

1.4.1.3 肺虚
1.4.1.3 Lung deficiency

主要表现:呼吸急促,声音低微,咳嗽声弱,自汗,舌淡,脉虚。

Main manifestations: Short and rapid breathing, feeble voice, weak and low sound of coughing, sweating on exertion, pale tongue, pulse of deficiency type.

1.4.1.4 肾虚
1.4.1.4 Kidney deficiency

主要表现:喘促日久,动则气促,喉间痰鸣,张口抬肩,气短倦怠,汗出,肢冷,舌质淡,脉沉细。

Main manifestations: dyspnea on exertion after longstanding asthma, severe wheezing, indrawing of the soft tisssues of the neck, short breath, lassitude and weakness, sweating, cold limbs, pale tongue, deep and thready pulse.

1.4.2 治疗
1.4.2 Treatment

1.4.2.1 风寒型
1.4.2.1 Wind cold
处方:肺俞、风门、大椎、列缺、合谷。
针以泻法并灸,以祛散风寒平喘。

Prescription:Feishu(BL 13),Fengmen(BL 12),Dazhui(DU 14),Lieque(LU 7),Hegu(LI 4).

Reducing method is applied in combination with moxibustion to eliminate wind cold and soothe asthma.

1.4.2.2 痰热型
1.4.2.2 Phlegm heat
处方:肺俞、定喘、天突、尺泽、丰隆。
针以泻法以清热化痰平喘。

Prescription:Feishu(BL 13),Dingchuan(EX—B 1),Tiantu(RN 22),Chize(LU 5),Fenglong(ST 40).

Acupuncture with reducing method to resolve phlegm, reduce heat and soothe asthma.

1.4.2.3 肺虚
1.4.2.3 Lung deficiency
处方:肺俞、太渊、足三里、太白。
针以补法或并灸,以补益肺气。

Prescription:Feishu(BL 13),Taiyuan(LU 9),Zusanli(ST 36),Taibai(SP 3).

Apply reinforcing method to strengthen the lung Qi. Moxibustion is also advisable.

1.4.2.4 肾虚
1.4.2.4 Kidney deficiency
处方:太溪、肾俞、肺俞、膻中、气海。
施以补法或并灸,补肾纳气。

持续喘息加身柱、膏肓俞;脾虚加中脘、脾俞。

Prescription: Taixi (KI 3), Shenshu (BL 23), Feishu (BL 13), Tanzhong (RN 17), Qihai (RN 6).

Reinforcing method is applied to strengthen the kidney function in receiving Qi. Moxibustion is also advisable.

For persistent asthma, plus Shenzhu (DU 12) and Gaohuang (BL 43); for the deficiency of spleen, plus Zhongwan (RN 12) and Pishu (BL 20).

该病包括支气管哮喘、喘息性支气管炎、阻塞性肺气肿以及其他疾病见有呼吸急促者。

This condition includes brochial asthma, asthmatic bronchitis, obstructive pulmonary emphysema and dyspnea present in some other diseases.

1.5 胃脘痛
1.5 Epigastric Pain

1.5.1 辨证
1.5.1 Differentiation

1.5.1.1 食积内停
1.5.1.1 Retention of food

主要表现:胃脘胀痛,按之或进食之后尤甚,嗳腐,纳呆,舌苔厚腻,脉滑有力。

Main manifestations: Distending pain in the epigastrium, aggravated on pressure or after meals, belching with fetid odour, anorexia, thick, sticky tongue coating, deep, forceful or rolling pulse.

1.5.1.2 肝气犯胃

1.5.1.2 Attack of the stomach by the stognant liver Qi

主要表现:胃脘阵痛,连及胁部,恶心嗳气,呕吐,吞酸,腹胀,厌食,舌苔薄白,脉沉弦。

Main manifestations:Paroxymal pain in the epigastrium, radiating to the hypochondriac regions, frequent belching accompanied by nausea, vomiting, acid regurgitation, abdominal distension, anorexia, thin, white tongue coating, deep, string—taut pulse.

1.5.1.3 胃虚有寒

1.5.1.3 Deficiency of the stomach with the accumulation of cold

主要表现:胃痛隐隐,得温得按痛减,倦怠疲乏,泛清水,舌苔薄白,脉沉迟。

Main manifestations:Dull pain in the epigastrium, which may be relieved by pressure and warmth, general lassitude, regurgitation of thin fluid, thin, white tongue coating, deep, slow pulse.

1.5.2 治疗
1.5.2 Treatment

1.5.2.1 食积内停
1.5.2.1 Retention of food

处方:建里、内关、足三里。
针以泻法消食和胃。

Prescription:Jianli(RN 11), Neiguan(PC 6), Zusanli(ST 36).

Acupuncture with reducing method to remove retention, pacify the stomach and relieve pain.

1.5.2.2 肝气犯胃

1.5.2.2 Attack of the stomach by the stagnant liver Qi

处方：期门、中脘、内关、足三里、太冲。

主要选取厥阴肝经及阳明胃经穴，针以泻法，以疏肝和胃止痛。

Prescription: Qimen(LR 14), Zhongwan(RN 12), Neiguan(PC 6), Zusanli(ST 36), Taichong(LR 3).

Points of Jueyin and Yangming channels of Foot are slected as the principal ones with the reducing method applied to remove the stangnation of liver Qi, to pacify the stomach and to relieve pain.

1.5.2.3 胃虚有寒
1.5.2.3 Deficiency of stomach with the accumulation of cold

处方：中脘、气海、脾俞、内关、足三里、公孙。

Prescription: Zhongwan(RN 12), Qihai(Rn 6), Pishu(BL 20), Neiguan(PC 6), Zusanli(ST 36), Gongsun(SP 4).

针灸并用以温中散寒、理气止痛。该症也可施以扶火罐疗法治疗。

Both acupuncture and moxibustion are used to warm up the middle jiao (middle warmer), dispel cold and regulate the flow of Qi and relieve pain. The cupping therapy is advisable in treatment of this disorder.

胃脘痛可见於现代医学之消化性溃疡、胃炎、胃神经官能症及胰腺、肝、胆疾病。

The epigastaric pain is a symptom found in petic ulcer, gastritis, gastric neurosis and diseases of the liver, gallbladder and pancreas in modern medicne.

1.6 呕吐
1.6 Vomiting

1.6.1 辨证
1.6.1 Differentiation

1.6.1.1 食积内停
1.6.1.1 Retention of food

主要表现:呕吐酸腐,脘腹胀满,嗳气,厌食,便溏或便秘,舌有腐苔,脉滑有力。

Main manifestation: Acid fermented vomitus, epigastric and abdominal distension, belching, anorexia, loose stool or constipation, thick granular tongue coating, rolling and forceful pulse.

1.6.1.2 肝气犯胃
1.6.1.2 Attack of the stomach by the stagnant liver Qi

主要表现:呕吐酸水,嗳气频频,胸胁胀痛,抑郁烦躁,舌苔薄腻,脉弦。

Main manifestations: Vomiting, acid regurgitation, frequent belching, distending pain in the chest and hypochondriac regions, irritability with an oppressed feeling, thin, slightly sticky tongue coating, string—taut pulse.

1.6.1.3 脾胃虚弱
1.6.1.3 Qi deficiency of the spleen and stomach

主要表现:面色萎黄,食后作呕,纳呆,倦怠疲乏,大便微溏,舌淡苔薄白,脉细无力。

Main manifestations: Sallow complexion, vomiting after a big meal, loss of appetite, lassitude, weakness, slightly loose stool, pale tongue, thin, white tongue coating, thready and forceless pulse.

1.6.2 治疗
1.6.2 Treatment

主要治则为降逆和胃。食积内停者针以泻法；肝胃不和者平补平泻法以调理气机；由于脾胃虚弱者当针以补法并灸以温中健脾和胃止呕。

处方：中脘、足三里、内关、公孙。

配穴：食积加下脘；肝气犯胃加太冲；脾胃虚弱加脾俞；持续呕吐加金津玉液。

The general principle of treatment is to activate the descent of Qi and to pacify the stomach. For the retention of food, reducing is indicated, for attack of stomach by the stagnant liver Qi, even method is used to soothe the liver and regulate the flow of Qi, and for weakness of the spleen and stomach, reinforcing combined with moxibustion is used to strengthen the function of spleen and warm up the middle warmer.

Prescription: Zhongwan (RN 12), Zusanli (ST 36), Neiguang (PC 6), Gongsun (SP 4).

Supplementary points:

Retention of food: Xiawan (RN 10); attack of the stomach by the liver Qi: Taichong (LR 3); weakness of the spleen and stomach: Pishu (BL 20); persistent vomiting: Jinjing and Yuye (EX-HN 12,13).

1.7 呃逆
1.7 Hiccup

1.7.1 辨证
1.7.1 Differentiation

1.7.1.1 食积内停
1.7.1.1 Retention of food

主要表现：呃声响亮，脘腹胀满，厌食，舌苔厚腻，脉滑有力。

Main manifestations: Loud hiccups, epigastric and abdominal distension, anorexia, thick, sticky tongue coating, rolling and forceful pulse.

1.7.1.2 气滞
1.7.1.2 Stagnation of Qi

主要表现：呃逆频频，胃脘胀痛，胸胁胀满，舌苔薄，脉弦有力。

Main manifestations: Continual hiccups, distending pain and feeling of oppression in the chest and in the hypochondrium, thin tongue coating, string—taut and forceful pulse.

1.7.1.3 胃寒
1.7.1.3 Cold in the stomach

主要表现：呃声沉缓有力，得温稍减，遇寒尤剧，胃脘不适，舌苔白润，脉迟。

Main manifestations: Slow and forceful hiccups which may be relieved by warmth and aggravated by cold, discomfort in the epigsatrium, white, moist tongue coating, slow pulse.

1.7.2 治疗
1.7.2 Treatment

主要治则为和胃降逆止呃,食积及气滞者针以泻法;胃寒者针灸并用以祛胃寒。

The principle of treatment is to pacify the stomach, to facilitate the descent of Qi and to check the hiccup. For the retention of food and stagnation of Qi, the reducing method should be applied; while for the cold in the stomach type, both acupuncture and moxibustion could be used to eliminate the cold evil.

处方:膈俞、中脘、内关、足三里。

食积加巨阙;气滞加膻中、太冲;胃寒者加上脘。

亦可用拔火罐治疗,常用穴位有:膈俞、膈关、肝俞、中脘和乳根。

Prescription: Geshu(BL 17), Zhongwan(RN 7), Neiguan(PC 6) and Zusanli(ST 36).

Supplementary points:

Retention of food: Juque(RN 14); stagnation of Qi: Tangzhong(RN 17) and Taichong(LR 3); For cold in the stomach, plus Shangwan(RN 13).

Cupping is also used in the treatment. Commonly used points are Geshu(BL 17), Geguan(BL 47), Ganshu(BL 18), Zhongwan(RN 12) and Rugen(ST 18).

1.8 腹痛
1.8 Abdominal Pain

1.8.1 辨证
1.8.1 Differentiation

1.8.1.1 寒邪腹痛
1.8.1.1 Accumulation of cold

主要表现:痛势急暴,喜温怕冷,大便溏薄,口淡不渴,小便清长,四肢不温,舌苔白,脉沉紧或弦紧。

Main manifestation: Sudden onset of violent abdominal pain which responds to warmth and gets worse by cold, loose stool, absence of thirst, clear and profuse urine, cold limbs, thin white tongue coating, deep and tense or string-taut and tense pulse.

1.8.1.2 脾阳不振
1.8.1.2 Hypoactivity of the spleen Yang

主要表现:腹痛缠绵,时作时止,痛时喜按,劳累、饥饿或遇寒加剧,神疲畏寒,苔薄白,脉沉细。

Main manifestation: Intermittent dull pain which may be relieved by warmth or by pressure and aggravated by cold or by hunger and fatigue, lassitude, aversion to cold, thin, white tongue coating, deep and thready pulse.

1.8.1.3 饮食停滞
1.8.1.3 Retention of food

主要表现:脘腹胀满,痛处拒按,恶食,嗳腐吞酸,或腹痛欲泄,泄后痛减,苔腻,脉滑。

Main manifestations: Epigastric and abdominal distending pain which is aggravated by pressure, anorexia, foul belching, and sour regurgitation, or abdominal pain accompanied by diarrhea and relieved after defecation, sticky coating, rolling pulse.

1.8.2 治疗
1.8.2 Treatment

1.8.2.1 寒邪腹痛
1.8.2.1 Accumulation of cold

处方:中脘、神阙、足三里、公孙。

针以泻法并灸以温里散寒。

Prescription: Zhongwan (RN 12), Shenque (RN 8), Zusanli (ST 36), Gongsun (SP 4).

Needle the points with the reducing method applied in combination with moxibustion to warm the stomach and dispel cold.

1.8.2.2 脾阳不振
1.8.2.2 Hypoactivity of the spleen Yang

处方:胃俞、脾俞、中脘、章门、气海、足三里。

针以补法并灸以温运脾胃之阳气。

Prescription: Weishu (BL 21), Pishu (BL 20), Zhongwan (RN 12) Zhangmen (LR 13), Qihai (RN 6), Zusanli (ST 36).

Acupuncture with reinforcing method and moxibustion are applied to warm and activate the spleen and stomach Yang.

1.8.2.3 饮食停滞
1.8.2.3 Retention of food

处方:中脘、天枢、气海、足三里。

针以泻法以消食导滞。

Prescription:Zhongwan(RN 12),Tianshu(ST 25),Qihai(RN 6), Zusanli(ST 36).

Apply acupuncturae with reducing method to remove the retention of food.

1.9 泄泻
1.9 Diarrhoea

1.9.1 辨证
1.9.1 Differentiation

1.9.1.1 急性泄泻
1.9.1.1 Acute diarrhoea

1.9.1.1.1 寒湿型

1.9.1.1.1 Cold—dampness

主要表现:水样泄,肠鸣腹痛,恶寒喜暖,口不渴,舌苔白,舌质淡,脉沉迟。

Main manifestations: Watery diarrhoea, abdominal pain and borborygmi, chillness which responds to warmth, absence of thirst, pale tongue, white tongue coating, deep and slow pulse.

1.9.1.1.2 湿热型

1.9.1.1.2 Damp heat

主要表现:腹痛泄泻,泻下黄糜热臭,肛门灼热,口渴,舌苔黄腻,脉滑数。

Main manifestations: Diarrhoea with abdominal pain, yellow hot

113

and fetid stools, burning sensation in the anus, scanty urine, or accompanied by general feverish feeling, thirst, yellow, sticky tongue coating, rolling and rapid pulse.

1.9.1.1.3 饮食内停

1.9.1.1.3 Retintion of food

主要表现:腹痛得泄则减,肠鸣,大便腐臭,脘腹胀满,嗳气厌食,舌苔厚浊,脉滑数或沉弦。

Main manifestations: Aabdominal pain relieved after bowel movements, borborygmi, diarrhoea with fetid stools, epigastric distension, belching and anorexia, thick granular tongue coating, rolling and rapid, or deep and string—taut pulse.

1.9.1.2 慢性泄泻

1.9.1.2 Chronic diarrhoea

1.9.1.2.1 脾虚

1.9.1.2.1 Deficiency of the spleen

主要表现:大便稀溏,水谷不化,纳呆,食后脘胀不适,神疲,面色萎黄,舌淡苔白,脉细无力。

Main manifestations: Loose stool with undigested food, anorexia, epigastric distress after eating, sallow complexion, lassitude, pale tongue, white tongue coating, thready, forceless pulse.

1.9.1.2.2 肾虚

1.9.1.2.2 Deficiency of the kidney

主要表现:脐下腹痛,肠鸣,五更泄泻,泄后痛减,遇寒加剧,时有腹胀,下肢不温,舌淡苔白,脉沉无力。

Main manifestations: Pain below the umbilicus, borborygmi, and diarrhoea usually occurring at dawn, relieved after bowel movements, and aggravated by cold, abdominal distension sometimes, cold lower extremities, pale tongue, white tongue coating, deep, forceless pulse.

1.9.2 治疗
1.9.2 Treatment

1.9.2.1 急性泄泻
1.9.2.1 Acute diarrhoea

选穴原则：主要选取足阳明胃经穴。

寒湿型者,针以泻法并隔姜灸以温中止泻；湿热者针以泻法清利湿热；食积者针以泻法以调和脾胃、消食导滞。

处方：天枢、足三里。

配穴：寒湿者加中脘、气海；湿热者加内庭、阴陵泉。

Principle of points selection: the points of the Yangming channel of Foot are selected as the principal ones.

Cold—dampness: Reducing method in combination with moxibustion (with ginger) is applied to warm the stomach and resolve the dampness.

Damp heat: Reducing is used to eliminate heat and dampness.

Retention of food: reducing is used to regulate the function of the spleen and stomach and remove stagnation.

Prescription: Tianshu(ST 25), Zusanli(ST 36).

Supplementary points:

Cold dampness: Zhongwan(RN 12), Qihai(RN 6).

Damp heat: Neiting (ST 44), Yinlingquan(SP 9).

1.9.2.2 慢性泄泻
1.9.2.2 Chronic diarrhoea

1.9.2.2.1 脾虚
1.9.2.2.1 Deficiency of spleen

处方：脾俞、章门、太白、中脘、足三里。

针以补法并灸以健脾止泻。

Prescription: Pishu(BL 20), Zhangmen(LR 13), Taibai(SP 3), Zhongwan(RN 12), Zusanli(ST 36).

Acupuncture with reinforcing and moxibustion are used to strengthen the function of spleen and to stop the diarrhoea.

1.9.2.2.2 肾虚

1.9.2.2.2 Deficiency of the kidney

处方:肾俞、脾俞、命门、关元、太溪、足三里。

选取督、任脉及肾经俞穴针以补法并灸以温肾壮阳。

Prescription: Shenshu(BL 23), Pishu(BL 20), Mingmen(DU 4), Guanyuan(RN 4), Taixi(KI 3), Zusanli (ST 36).

The points of the Kidney channel, Ren and Du meridians are selected as the principal points with the reinforcing method and moxibustion to warm and reinforce the kidney Yang.

该病包括现代医学之急慢性肠炎、消化不良、肠道寄生虫病、胰腺及肝胆疾病、内分泌及代谢紊乱以及神经官能症等。

This condition may be involved in acute and chronic enteritis, indigestion, intestinal parasitic diseases, diseases of the pancreas, liver and biliary tract, endocrine and metabolic disorders, and neurotic troubles.

1.10 腹胀
1.10 Abdominal Distention

1.10.1 辨证
1.10.1 Differentiation

1.10.1.1 实证
1.10.1.1 Excess condition

主要表现:持续腹部胀满,腹痛拒按,口臭,尿黄便秘,有时可见发热,呕吐,舌苔黄腻,脉滑数有力。

Main manifestations: Persistence of distention and fullness in abdomen, which is aggravated by pressure, abdominal pain, belching, foul breath, dark yelllow urine, constipation, sometimes associated with fever, vomiting, yellow thick tongue coating, rolling, rapid and forceful pulse.

1.10.1.2 虚证
1.10.1.2 Deficiency condition

主要表现:腹胀喜按,肠鸣,便溏,纳减,神倦疲乏,尿清,舌淡苔白,脉弱。

Main manifestations: Abdominal distention relieved by pressure, borborygmi, loose stools, loss of appetite, lassitude, listlessness, clear urine, pale tongue with white coating and forceless pulse.

1.10.2 治疗
1.10.2 Treatment

处方:中脘、天枢、足三里、上巨虚。

配穴:实证加合谷、阴陵泉;虚证加关元、太白。

实证针以泻法以调通腑气;虚证施以补法并灸以补益脾胃、理气消胀。

Prescription: Zhongwan (RN 12), Tianshu(ST 25), Zusanli(ST 36) and Shangjuxu(ST 37).

Supplementary points:

Excess condition: Hegu(LI 4), Qihai(RN 6), Yinlingquan(SP

9).

Deficiency condition: Guanyuan(Rn 4), Taibai(SP 4).

The excess condition is treated by the reducing method to regulate the Qi flow in the Fu organs while the deficiency condition is treated with the reinforcing method or combined with moxibustion to invigorate the function of spleen and stomach and to adjust the circulation of Qi to relieve the distention.

该病包括现代医学之胃下垂、急性胃扩张、肠麻痹、急性肠梗阻、胃肠神经官能症等。

This condition is involved in gastroptosis, acute gastrectasia, enteroparalysis, intestinal obstruction, gastrointestinal neurosis, etc.

1.11 便秘
1.11 Constipation

1.11.1 辨证
1.11.1 Differentiation

1.11.1.1 实秘
1.11.1.1 Excess condition

主要表现：便次减少，三、五日一次或更长时间。如属热邪壅结，则见身热、烦渴、口臭、脉滑有力、舌苔黄干；气机郁滞者则见胁腹胀满或疼痛、嗳气频作、纳食减少、舌苔薄腻、脉弦。如阴寒凝结则见腹中冷痛，喜热畏寒，舌质淡，苔白润，脉沉迟。

Main manifestations: Infrequent and difficult defecation from every three to five days, or even longer. In case of accumulation of heat, there are fever, thirst, foul breath, rolling and forceful pulse, yellow, dry tongue coating; in case of stagnation of Qi there are fullness and distending pain in the abdomen and hypochondriac regions, frequent belching, loss of appetite, thin sticky tongue coating and string—taut pulse. In cases of accumulation of cold, pain and cold sesation in the abdomen, preference for warmth and aversion to cold, pale tongue with white and moist coating, deep slow pulse.

1.11.1.2 虚秘
1.11.1.2 Deficiency condition

主要表现:便秘如因气血虚者则面色唇爪胱白无华,头晕心悸,神疲气怯,舌淡苔薄,脉细弱。

Main manifestations: In cases of deficiency of Qi and Blood, pale and lustreless complexion, lips and nails, dizziness and palpitation, lassitude, shortness of breath, pale tongue with thin coating, thready and weak pulse.

1.11.2 治疗
1.11.2 Treatment

实秘泻之以清热通便,理气通便或温通腑气而通便;虚秘补之以补益气血,润肠通便。

处方:大肠俞、天枢、支沟、照海。

热结者配以曲池、合谷;气滞者加太冲、中脘;气血不足加脾俞、胃俞、足三里;寒凝者加灸神阙、气海。

For the excess condition the reducing method is applied to eliminate the heat, moisten the intestine, and remove the stagnation of Qi, Constipation due to cold can be relieved by moxibustion to warm the Fu organ for defecation; while for deficiency condition, the reinforcing method is used to reinforce Qi and blood, and moisten the intestines for defecation.

Prescription: Dachangshu(BL 25), Tianshu(ST 25), Zhigou(SJ 6), Zhaohai (KI 6).

Accumulation of heat: Quchi(LI 11), Hegu(LI 4).

Stagnation of Qi: Zhongwan(RN 12), Taichong(LR 3).

Deficiency of Qi and blood: Pishu(BL 20), Weishu(BL 21), Zusanli(ST 36).

Agglomeration of cold: Moxibustion to Shenque(RN 8) and Qihai (RN 4).

1.12 脱肛
1.12 Prolapse of Rectum

1.12.1 辨证
1.12.1 Differentiation

主要表现:起病缓慢,起始肛门排便有胀坠感,便后正常。如未治疗,稍有劳累即发,垂脱后收摄无力,须以手助其回纳,或兼见神疲肢软,面色萎黄,头眩心悸等症,舌淡苔白,脉多濡细。

Main manifestations: The onset is slow, to start with distending and draggling sensation of rectum during defecation, and returning to normal after the bowel movement. If it is sustained without proper treatment, recurrence may happen by overstrain and the prolapsed rectum fails to return spontaneously without the aid of the hand.

Sometimes there are lassitude, weakness of limbs, sallow complexion, dizziness and palpitation. The tongue is pale with white coating, and the pulse thready and feeble.

1.12.2 治疗
1.12.2 Treatment

针以补法并灸。
处方:百会、大肠俞、长强、足三里。
Apply the acupuncture with reinforcing method and moxibustion.
Prescription: Baihui(DU 20), Dachangshu(BL 25), Changqiang (DU 1), Zusanli(ST 36).

1.13 水肿
1.13 Edema

1.13.1 辨证
1.13.1 Differentiation

1.13.1.1 阳水
1.13.1.1 Yang edema

主要表现:急性起病,初起面目微肿,继则遍及全身,皮肤光泽伴见发热恶寒,口渴,咳嗽气喘,尿量减少,舌苔薄白,脉浮滑而数。

Main manifestations: Abrupt onset of edema with puffy face and eyelids and then anasarca, lustrous skin, accompanied by chills, fever, thirst, cough, asthma and reduced urine output, thin white tongue coating, superficial or rolling, rapid pulse.

1.13.1.2 阴水

1.13.1.2 Yin edema

主要表现:由渐而始,初起眼睑或足跗微肿,继而肿遍全身,而以腰以下尤甚;伴见面色萎黄,恶寒肢冷,腰部酸痛,全身无力,脘腹胀满,纳食减少,大便溏,舌质淡苔白,脉沉细。

Main manifestations: Insidious onset of edema, at first on the pedis dorsum or eyelids, and then over the whole body, especially remarkable below the lumbar region, aaccompanied by sallow complexion, aversion to cold, cold limbs, sorness of the back and loins, general weakness, epigastric fullness, abdominal distension, loss of appetite, loose stools, pale tongue, white coating, deep, thready pulse.

1.13.2 治疗

1.13.2 Treatment

1.13.2.1 阳水

1.13.2.1 Yang edema

处方:列缺、合谷、偏历、阴陵泉、委阳。

针以平补平泻法以宣肺解表,利水消肿。表证解后按阴水诊治。

Prescription: Lieque(LU 7), Hegu(LI 4), Pianli(LI 6) Yinlingquan(SP 9), Weiyang(BL 39).

Apply the even method to clear the lung, relieve the exterior symptoms and remove the retained fluid. After the exterior symptoms are relieved, refer to method for Yin edema.

1.13.2.2 阴水

1.13.2.2 Yin edema

处方:脾俞、肾俞、水分、关元、复溜、足三里。

配穴:面肿加水沟;足背肿加足临泣、商丘。

针施以补法加灸。

Prescription: Pishu(BL 20), Shenshu(BL 23), Shuifen(RN 9) Guanyuan(RN 4), Fuliu(KI 7), Zusanli(ST 36).

Supplementary points:

Facial puffiness: Shuigou(DU 26).

Edema on the pedis dorsum: Zulinqi(GB 41), Shanqiu(SP 5).

Treat the patient with reinforcing method and moxibustion.

1.14 遗尿
1.14 Nocturnal Enuresis

1.14.1 辨证
1.14.1 Differentiation

主要表现:夜间遗尿,轻者数夜一次,重者一夜数次,面色萎黄,纳呆,久病者体弱,舌淡苔白,尺部脉弱。

Main manifestations: Involuntary micturition during sleep with dreams, once in several nights in mild cases, or several times a night in severe cases; sallow complexsion, loss of appetite, and weakness in the prolonged cases, pale tongue, white coating, thready pulse weak at the Chi region.

1.14.2 治疗
1.14.2 Treatment

处方:肾俞、膀胱俞、中极、三阴交、大敦。

配穴:有梦遗尿加神门针以补法并灸。纳呆加脾俞、足三里。

Prescription: Shenshu(BL 23), Pangguangshu(BL 28), Zhongji (RN 3), Sanyinjiao(SP 6), Dadun(LR 1). Needle the Points with reinforcing method and apply moxibustion.

Supplementaray points:

Euresis with dreams: Shenmen(HT 7);

Loss of appetite: Pishu(BL 20), Zusanli(ST 36).

该病主要原因是大脑皮层排尿中枢发育不完善,针灸疗法效果较好。如遗尿是由器质性疾病如尿道畸形、隐性脊柱裂、脑部器质性病变以及蛲虫等,须积极治疗原发病。

The chief causative factor of this disorder is the underdevelopment of cerebral micturition centre and treatment of acupuncture and moxibustion provides satisfactory effect. As for enuresis caused by organic diseases such as, deformity of urinary tract, cryptorachischisis, organic cerebral diseases and oxyuriasis, the treatment should be given to the primary disease.

1.15 淋证
1.15 Urination Disturbance

1.15.1 辨证
1.15.1 Differentiation

1.15.1.1 石淋
1.15.1.1 Dysuria caused by calculi

主要表现:尿中偶有砂石,排尿困难,尿短赤而浊,或排尿突然中断,腰腹疼痛,排尿刺痛难忍,或尿中有血。

Main manifestations: Occasional presence of calculi in the urine, dysuria, dark yellow turbid urine, or sudden interruption of urination, unberable pricking pain during urination, pain of the lumbus and abdomen, or presence of blood in the urine.

1.15.1.2 气淋

1.15.1.2 Dysuria caused by Qi dysfunction

主要表现:排尿滴沥不爽,下腹胀痛,舌苔薄白,脉沉弦。

Main manifestations: Difficult and hesitant urination, fullness and pain of the lower abdomen, thin, white tongue coating, deep string—taut pulse.

1.15.1.3 血淋

1.15.1.3 Painful urination with blood

主要表现:血尿,尿痛,尿急,排尿时有热感、刺痛难忍,舌苔薄黄,脉数有力。

Main manifestations: Hematuria with pain and urgency of micturition, burning sensation and pricking pain in urination, thin, yellow tongue coating, rapid, forceful pulse.

1.15.1.4 膏淋

1.15.1.4 Dysuria with milky urine

主要表现:小便混浊,如膏如脂,尿道灼痛,舌红苔黄,脉细数。

Main manifestations: Cloudy urine with milky or creamy appearance, urethral burning pain in urination, red tongue proper, sticky coation, thready, rapid pulse.

1.15.1.5 劳淋

1.15.1.5 Dysuria caused by overstrain

主要表现:小便困难,滴沥不尽,时发时止,过劳则甚,常常久治难愈,脉弱。

Main manifestations: Difficulty in urination with dribbling of urine, occurring off and on, exacerbated after overwork, and usually refractory to teatment, weak pulse.

1.15.2 治疗
1.15.2 Treatment

按实则泻之；虚则补之，可灸
处方：膀胱俞、中极、阴陵泉。
加减：石淋，排尿困难加委阳；气淋小便不畅加行间；尿痛、血尿加血海、三阴交；膏淋尿如膏脂加肾俞、照海；劳淋加气海、百会、足三里。

Treat the difficient syndromes with reinforcing, and the excessive syndromes with reducing. Moxibustion is applicable.

Prescription: Pangguangshu (BL 28), Zhongji (RN 3), Yinlingquan (SP 9).

Supplementary points:

Dysura caused by calcluli: Weiyang (BL 39).

Dysuria caused by Qi dysfunction: Xingjian (LR 2).

Painful urination with blood: Xuehai (SP 10), Sanyinjiao (SP 6).

Dysuria with milky urine: Shenshu (BL 23), Zhaohai (KI 6).

Dysuria caused by overstrain: Baihui (DU 20), Qihai (RN 6), Zusanli (ST 36).

该病包括现代医学之尿路感染和泌尿系结石。

This condition includes urinary infection and urolithiasis in modern medicine.

1.16 癃闭
1.16 Retention of Urine

1.16.1 辨证
1.16.1 Differentiation

1.16.1.1 热结膀胱
1.16.1.1 Accumulation of heat in the bladder

主要表现：尿少灼热或尿闭，下腹胀满，口渴不欲饮，便秘，舌红苔黄，脉数。

Main manifestations: Scanty hot urine or retention of urine, distension and fullness of the lower abdomen, thirst but without desire to drink, constipation, red tongue with yellow coating, rapid pulse.

1.16.1.2 肾阳虚衰
1.16.1.2 Decline of Kidney Yang

主要表现：尿有余沥，排尿无力，面色㿠白，倦怠无力，下肢冷，腰膝酸软，舌质淡，脉沉细，尺部无力。

Main manifestations: Dribbling urination, decreasing in force of the urine discharge, pale complexion, listlessness, chilliness below the lumbus, weakness of the loins and knees, pale tongue, deep, thready pulse, weak at the Chi region.

1.16.1.3 气机阻滞
1.16.1.3 Stagnation of Qi

主要表现：小便滴沥不尽或尿闭，下腹隐隐胀痛，舌有瘀点，脉涩而数。

Main manifestations: Dribbling urination or retention of urine, distension and dull pain in the lower abdomen, purplish spots on the tongue, hesitant, rapid pulse.

1.16.2 治疗
1.16.2 Treatment

1.16.2.1 热结膀胱
1.16.2.1 Accumulation of heat in the bladder
处方:膀胱俞、中极、三阴交、委阳。
施以泻法以清热利尿。

Prescription: Pangguanshu (BL 28), Zhongji (Rn 3), Sanyinjiao (SP 6), Weiyang (BL 39).

Reducing method is applied to remove the heat and promote diuresis.

1.16.2.2 肾阳虚衰
1.16.2.2 Decline of Kidney Yang
处方:命门、肾俞、百会、关元、阳池。
施以补法或灸法以温肾壮阳。

Prescription: Mingmen (Du 4), Shenshu (BL 23), Baihui (DU 20), Guanyuan (RN 4), Yangchi (SJ 4).

Reinforcing or moxibustion is applied to warm the kidney yang.

1.16.2.3 气机阻滞
1.16.2.3 Stagnation of Qi
选取膀胱募穴为主穴,施以平补平泻法疏调气机、通利膀胱。
处方:中极、三阴交、水道、水泉。

The Front-(Mu) point of the bladder is selected as the principle point. Even method is applied to promote circulation of the Qi in the meridian and restore the function of the bladder.

Prescription: Zhongji(Rn 3), Sanyinjiao(SP 6), Shuidao(ST 28), Shuiquan(KI 5).

1.17 阳痿
1.17 Impotence

1.17.1 辨证
1.17.1 Differentiation

1.17.1.1 肾阳虚衰
1.17.1.1 Decline of Kidney Yang

主要表现：阳痿不举或举而不坚,面色㿠白,四肢冷,头晕倦怠,腰膝酸软,尿频,舌淡苔白脉沉细。心脾气虚者可兼见心悸,失眠。

Main manifestations: Failure of the penis in erection, weak erection, pallor, cold extremities, dizziness, listlessness, soreness and weakness of the loins and knees, frequent urination, pale tongue with white coating, deep thready pulse. If the heart and spleen Qi is damaged, palpitations and insomnia my be present.

1.17.1.2 湿热下注
1.17.1.2 Downward flowing of damp heat

主要表现：阳痿不举,兼见口苦口干,小便灼赤,下肢酸软,舌苔黄腻,脉濡数。

Main manifestations: Inability of the penis to erect, complicated with bitter taste in the mouth, thirst, hot and dark red urine, sorness and weakness of the lower extremities, yellow, sticky tongue coating, soft, rapid pulse.

1.17.2 治疗
1.17.2 Treatment

1.17.2.1 肾阳虚衰
1.17.2.1 Decline of Kidney Yang

处方:关元、命门、肾俞、太溪。

施以补法和灸法以温补肾阳;兼见心脾气虚者加针心俞、神门、三阴交。

Prescription: Guanyuan (Rn 4), Mingmen (DU 4), Shenshu (BL 23), Taixi (KI 3).

Reinforcing method with moxibustion is applied to invigorate the kidney yang.

supplementary points:

For damage of the Qi of the heart and spleen: Xinshu (BL 15), Shenmen (HT 7), Sanyinjiao (SP 6).

1.17.2.2 湿热下注
1.17.2.2 Downward flowing of damp heat

处方:中极、三阴交、阴陵泉、足三里。

施以泻法以清利湿热。

Prescription: Zhongji (RN 3), Sanyinjiao (SP 6), Yinlingquan (SP 9), Zusanli (ST 36).

Reducing method is applied to eliminate the damp heat.

1.18 失眠
1.18 Insomnia

1.18.1 辨证
1.18.1 Differentiation

1.18.1.1 心脾两虚
1.18.1.1 Deficiency of both the heart and spleen Qi

主要表现：入睡困难，多梦，心悸健忘，倦怠疲乏，面色萎黄，纳呆，舌淡苔薄，脉来细弱。

Main manifestations: Difficulty in falling asleep, dream-disturbed sleep, palpitation, poor memory, lassitude, listlessness, anorexia, sallow complexion, pale tongue with a thin coating, thready, weak pulse.

1.18.1.2 心肾不交
1.18.1.2 Disharmony between the heart and kidney

主要表现：烦躁不眠，头晕耳鸣，口干咽燥，五心烦热，舌红脉细数；或梦遗，健忘，心悸，腰酸痛。

Main manifestations: Restlessness, insomnia, dizziness, tinnitus, dry mouth with little saliva, burning sensation of the chest, palms and soles, red tongue, thready rapid pulse, or nocturnal emission, poor memory, palpitation, low back pain.

1.18.1.3 肝火上炎
1.18.1.3 Upward disturbance of the liver fire

主要表现：难以入睡，烦躁易怒，多梦，心惊易怯；兼见头痛，胁胀，口苦，脉弦。

Main manifestations: Difficulty in falling into sleep, irritability, dream-disturbed sleep, fright and fear accompanied with headache, distending pain in the costal region, bitter taste in the mouth and string-taut pulse.

1.18.1.4 胃气不和

1.18.1.4 **Dysfunction of the stomach**

主要表现:失眠,胃脘胀痛,痞闷不适,呃逆,或排便不畅,苔腻,脉滑。

Main manifestations: Insomnia, suffocating feeling and distending pain in the epigastric region, belching, or difficult defecation, sticky tongue coating, and rolling pulse.

1.18.2 治疗

1.18.2 Treatment

主要选取心经穴位以安神定志。心脾两虚者,补法和灸法并用以补益心脾;心肾不交者平补平泻以交通心肾;肝火上炎者施以泻法以清泻肝火;胃气不和者施以泻法以和胃安神。

处方:神门、三阴交。

心脾两虚者加针心俞、脾俞、隐白;

心肾不交者加针心俞、神门、太溪;

肝火上炎者加针肝俞、胆俞、完骨;

胃气不和者加针胃俞、足三里。

Points of heart meridian are selectled as the main points to calm the heart and soothe the mind.

Deficiency of the heart and spleen: Reinforcing method with moxibustion in combination is applied to strengthen the heart and spleen.

Disharmony between the heart and kidney: Even method is applied to harmonize the heart and kidney.

Upward disturbance of the liver fire: Reducing is applied to subdue the liver fire.

Dysfunction of the stomach: Reducing method is applied to regulatte the stomach Qi.

Prescription: Shenmen (HT 7), Sanyinjiao(SP 6).

Supplementary Points:

Deficiency of the heart and spleen: Pishu (BL 20), Xinshu (BL 15), Yinbai(SP 1).

Disharmony between the heart and kidney: Xinshu(BL 15), Shenshu(BL 23), Taixi(KI 3).

Upward disturbance of liver fire: Ganshu (BL 18), Danshu (BL 19), Wangu(GB 12).

Dysfunction of the stomach: Weishu(BL 21), Zusanli(ST 36)

1.19 心悸
1.19 Palpitation

1.19.1 辨证
1.19.1 Differentiation

1.19.1.1 心虚胆怯
1.19.1.1 Deficiency of heart and gallbladder

主要表现：心悸不宁，惊慌易恐，烦躁易怒，多梦，纳呆，舌苔薄白，脉稍数；有痰热内阻者，舌苔黄腻，脉滑数。

Main manifestations: Palpitation, fear and fright, irritability, restlessness, dream-disturbed sleep, anorexia, white, thin tongue coating, slightly rapid pulse. In cases of phlegm heat, yellow, sticky tongue coating, rolling, rapid pulse.

1.19.1.2 气血不足
1.19.1.2 Insufficiency of Qi and blood

主要表现：心悸，面色无华，头晕眼花，倦怠气短，舌淡有齿印，脉细弱或不齐。

Main manifestations: Palpitation, lustreless complexion, dizziness, blurring of vision, shortness of breath, lassitude, pale tongue with teeth prints, thready, weak or intermittent pulse.

1.19.1.3 阴虚火旺
1.19.1.3 Fire hyperactivity due to Yin deficiency

主要表现：心悸，烦躁易怒，失眠，头晕眼花，耳鸣，舌红少苔，脉来细数。

Main manifestations: Palpitation, restlessness, irritability, insomnia, dizziness, blurring of vision, tinnitus, red tongue with little coating, thready, rapid pulse.

1.19.1.4 痰饮内停
1.19.1.4 Rentention of pathogenic fluid and phlegm

主要表现：心悸，咳吐痰涎，胸脘痞闷，肢体倦怠，四肢冷，舌苔白，脉弦滑。脾肾阳虚者，兼有尿少，口干不欲饮，舌苔白滑，脉沉。

Main manifestations: Palpitation, expectoration of mucoid sputum, fullness in the chest and epigastric region, lassitude, weakness, cold extremities, white tongue coating, string-taut, rolling pulse. In case of deficiency of Yang in the spleen and kidney, decreased output of urine, thirst without desire to drink, white, slippery tongue coating, deep, string-taut or rapid pulse.

1.19.2 治疗
1.19.2 Treatment

选取心之背俞及募穴,心经的俞穴为主。对心虚胆怯者施平补平泻以宁心安神定志;气血不足者施以补法以养心益气安神;对阴虚火旺者,补泻并用以滋阴泻火;痰饮内停者先以泻法后施补法及灸法以温阳化痰饮。

处方:心俞、巨阙、神门、内关。

心虚胆怯加通里、丘墟;兼有痰热再加丰隆、胆俞;气血不足加脾俞、胃俞、足三里;阴虚火旺者加厥阴俞、肾俞、太溪;痰饮内停者加水分、关元、神阙、阴陵泉。

本篇所列心悸包括现代医学中的迷走神经功能失调及各种原因引起的心律失常的心悸。

The back-(Shu) and Front-(Mu) points of the heart, and points of the Heart and Pericardium Meridians are selected as the main ones. Even manipulation is applied for deficiency of heart and gallbladder to calm the heart. Reinforcing is used for insufficiency of Qi and blood to nourish the heart and ease the mind. Reinforcing combined with reducing is applied for fire hyperactiviry due to Yin deficiency to nourish Yin and subdue the fire. For retention of pathogenic fluid, reducing is applied first and then reinforcing in combination with moxibustion to warm Yang and dissolve the pathogenic fluid.

Prescription: Xinshu(Bl 15), Juque(RN 14), Shenmen(HT 7), Neiguan(PC 6).

Supplementary points:

Deficiency of heart and gallbladder: Tongli(PC 5), Qiuxu (GB 40); if accompanied with phlegm heat: Fenglong(ST 40), Danshu(BL

19). Insufficiency of Qi and blood: Pishu(BL 20), Weishu(BL 21), Zusanli(ST 36).

Fire hyperactivity due to Yin deficiency: Jueyinshu(BL 14), Shenshu(BL 23), Taixi (KI 3).

Retention of pathogenic fluid and phlegm: Shuifen (RN 9), Guanyuan(RN 4), Shenque(RN 8), Yinlingquan(SP 9).

Palpitation described here may be involved in neurosis, functional disorders of the vegetative nervous system and cardiac arrhythmia of various origins.

1.20 癫痫
1.20 Epilepsy

1.20.1 辨证
1.20.1 Differentiation

1.20.1.1 发作期
1.20.1.1 During seizure

主要表现:典型的癫痫发作往往起始有头晕,头痛,以及窒息感;继而突然仆倒,神志丧失,面色苍白,牙关紧闭,双眼上视,抽搐,口吐泡沫,口作猪羊叫声,甚至二便失禁。渐而病人神志清醒,诸症消失。除了疲劳之外,病人正常生活。舌苔白腻,脉弦滑。

Main manifestations: A typical seizure is preceded by dizziness, headache and suffocating sensation in the chest, and immediately followed by falling down with loss of consciousness, pallor, clenched jaws, upward staring of the eyes, convulsion, foam on the lips, screaming as pigs or sheep, and even incontinence of urine and feces. Gradually, the patient regains consciouseness, and the symptoms dissappear. Apart from fatigue and weakness, the patient can live a normal life. White sticky tongue coating, and string-taut, rolling pulse.

1.20.1.2 发作后
1.20.1.2 After seizure

主要表现:疲乏无力,面色无华,头晕,心悸,纳呆,痰多,腰膝酸软,舌淡苔白,脉滑细。

Main manifestations: Listlessness, lustreless complexion, dizziness, palpitation, anorexia, profuse sputum, weakness and soreness of the loins and limbs, pale tongue with white coating and thready, rolling pulse.

1.20.2 治疗
1.20.2 Treatment

1.20.2.1 发作期
1.20.2.1 During seizure

处方:水沟、鸠尾、间使、太冲、丰隆。

主要选取任、督及肝经穴位,施以泻法以涤痰开窍醒神,平肝熄风。

Prescription: Shuigou(DU 26), Jiuwei(RN 15), Jianshi(PC 5), Taichong(LR 3), Fenglong(ST 40).

Points of the Du, Ren and liver meridians are selected with reducing method to dissolve the phlegm, induce resuscitation, soothe the liver and dispel the wind.

1.20.2.2 发作后
1.20.2.2 After seizure

主要选取心、脾、肾经俞穴,施以平补平泻法以宁心安神,健脾益肾。

处方：心俞、印堂、神门、三阴交、太溪、腰奇。

加减：日间发作者加申脉；夜间发作加照海；痰郁者加中脘、丰隆；气血亏虚者加关元、足三里。

Points of the heart, spleen and kidney meridians are selected as the main ones with even method to nourish the heart, ease the mind, strengthen the spleen and reinforce the kidney.

Prescription: Xinshu(BL 15), Yintang(EX-HN 3), Shenmen(HT 7), Sanyinjiao(SP 6), Taixi(KI 3), Yaoqi (EX-B 9).

Supplementary points:

Daytime seizure: Shemnai (BL 62).

Night seizure: Zhaohai(KI 6).

Phlegm stagnation: Zhongwan(JN 12), Fenglong(ST 40).

Severe deficiency of Qi and blood: Guanyuan(RN 4), Zusanli(ST 36).

本篇所论包括各种类型的癫痫发作，包括癫痫大发作、小发作、精神运动性发作及局限性发作。对于继发性癫痫，应积极治疗原发病。

The above description refers to many types of epileptic seizures including grand mal, petit mal, psychomotor and focal seizures. For secondary epilepsy, the primary disease should be treated actively.

1.21 头晕
1.21 Dizziness

1.21.1 辨证
1.21.1 Differentiation

1.21.1.1 肝阳上亢
1.21.1.1 Hyperactivity of Liver Yang

主要表现：头晕，怒时尤甚，烦躁，目红面赤，耳鸣，口苦，多梦，舌质红苔黄，脉弦数。

Main manifestations: Dizziness aggravated by anger, irritability, flushed face, red eyes, tinnitus bitter taste in the mouth, dream-disturbed sleep, red tongue proper with yellow coating, string-taut, rapid pulse.

1.21.1.2 气血两虚
1.21.1.2 Deficiency of Qi and blood

主要表现：面色苍白无华，头晕，倦怠，心悸失眠，唇甲苍白。头晕多发于重病或失血之后，劳累后加剧，重者可有昏倒。

Main manifestations: Dizziness accompanied by pallor and lustreless complexion, weakness, palpitation, insomnia, pale lips and nails, lassitude, pale tongue proper, thready and weak pulse. Dizziness occurs mostly after a serious disease or loss of blood and is aggravated by overwork. Syncope happens in severe cases.

1.21.1.3 痰湿内停
1.21.1.3 Interior retention of phlegm dampness

主要表现：头晕头重，胸闷不适，恶心痰多，纳呆嗜睡，舌苔白腻,脉濡滑。

Main manifestations: Dizziness with a heavy feeling of the head and suffocating sensation in the chest, nausea, profuse sputum, anorexia, somonlence, white, sticky tongue coating, soft, rolling pulse.

1.21.2 治疗
1.21.2 Treatment

1.21.2.1 肝阳上亢
1.21.2.1 Hyperactivity of Liver Yang
处方:风池、肝俞、肾俞、太溪、行间。
施以补泻并用,孰先孰后视病情而定。

Prescription: Fengchi (GB 20), Ganshu (BL 18), Shenshu (BL 23), Taixi(KI 3), Xingjian(LR 2).

Reinforcing and reducing methods are applied with either one first according to the condition of the disease.

1.21.2.2 气血两虚
1.21.2.2 Deficiency of Qi and blood
处方:百会、脾俞、关元、足三里、三阴交。
施以补法及灸法以滋补气血。

Prescription: Baihui(DU 20), Pishu(BL 20), Guanyuan(RN 4), Zusanli (ST 36), Sanyinjiao(SP 6).

Apply reinforcing method combined with moxibustion to replenish Qi and blood.

1.21.2.3 痰湿内停
1.21.2.3 Interior retention of phlegm dampness
处方:头维、脾俞、中脘、内关、丰隆。
施以泻法以祛痰除湿。

Prescription: Touwei(ST 8), Pisu(BL 20), Zhongwan(RN 12), Neiguan(PC 6), Fenglong(ST 40).

Apply even method to resolve phlegm and eliminate dampness.

1.22 郁证
1.22 Melancholia

1.22.1 辨证
1.22.1 Differentiation

1.22.1.1 肝气郁结
1.22.1.1 Depression of the Qi in the liver

主要表现:情志抑郁,胸闷不适,胁痛腹胀,呃逆纳呆或腰痛,呕吐,舌苔白腻,脉弦。

Main manifestations: Mental depression, distress of the chest, hypochondriac pain, abdominal distension, belching, anorexia, abdominal pain, vomiting, thin, sticky tongue coating, string-taut pulse.

1.22.1.2 气郁化火
1.22.1.2 Transformation of depressed Qi into fire

主要表现:头痛,口苦口干,烦躁胸闷,胁胀,吞酸,便秘,耳鸣目赤,舌红苔黄,脉弦数。

Main manifestations: Headache, dryness and bitter taste in the mouth, irritability, distress of the chest, hypochondriac distension, acid regurgitation, constipation, red eyes, tinnitus, red tongue with yellow coating, string-taut, rapid pulse.

1.22.1.3 痰郁

1.22.1.3　Stagnation of phlegm

主要表现:喉中有如异物梗阻,吞之不下,吐之不出,薄腻苔,脉弦滑。

Main manifestations: Feeling of a lump choking in the throat, hard to spit it out or to swallow it, thin, sticky tongue coating, string-taut, rolling pulse.

1.22.1.4　血虚（癔病）

1.22.1.4　Insufficiency of blood (hysteria)

主要表现:悲伤善哭,喜怒无常,多疑善恐,心悸,易怒,失眠;或突觉胸闷,呃逆,或突然不语,甚则抽搐或意识丧失;苔薄白,脉弦细。

Main manifestations: Grief without reasons, caprecious joy or anger, suspicious, liability to get frightened, palpitation, irritability, insomnia, or sudden distress of the chest, hiccup, sudden aphonia, convulsion, or loss of consciousness in severe cases, thin, white tongue coating, string-taut, thready pulse.

1.22.2　治疗

1.22.2　Treatment

1.22.2.1　肝气郁结

1.22.2.1　Depression of Qi in the liver

处方:肝俞、膻中、中脘、足三里、公孙、太冲。

施以平补平泻以疏肝理脾,调和胃气。

Prescription: Ganshu(BL 18), Tanzhong(Rn 17), Zhongwan(kRN 12), Zusanli (St 36), Gongsun(SP 4), Taichong(LR 3).

Even method is applied to soothe the liver, strengthen the spleen and harmonize the stomach.

1.22.2.2 气郁化火

1.22.2.2 **Transformation of depressed Qi into fire**

处方:上脘、支沟、阳陵泉、行间、侠溪。

施以泻法以泻肝火,调胃气。

Prescription: Shangwan (RN 13), Zhigou (SJ 6), Yanglingquan (GB 34), Xingjian(LR 2), Xiaxi(GB 43).

Reducing method is used to dispel the fire form the liver and strengthen the stomach function.

1.22.2.3 痰郁

1.22.2.3 **Stagnation of phlegm**

处方:天突、膻中、内关、丰隆、太冲。

施以平补平泻以疏肝解郁,理气除痰。

Prescription: Tiantu (RN 22), Tanzhong (RN 17), Neiguan (PC 6), Fenglong(ST 40), Taichong(LR 3).

Even method is used to soothe the liver, remove the depression, regulate the flow of Qi and resolve phlegm.

1.22.2.4 血虚(癔病)

1.22.2.4 **Insufficiency of blood(hysteria)**

主要选取心、肝经俞穴,平补平泻以养血柔肝,安神定志。

处方:巨阙、神门、三阴交、太冲。

加减配穴:

胸闷加针内关、膻中;

呃逆加针公孙、天突;

突然不语加针通里、廉泉;

抽搐加针合谷、阳陵泉;

神志不清加针水沟、涌泉。

Points of the heart and liver meridians are selected as the principal points. Even method is applied to nourish blood, soothe the liver and refresh and tranquilize the mind.

Prescription: Juque(RN 14), Shenmen(HT 7), Sanyinjiao(SP 6), Taichong(LR 3),

Supplementary points:

Distress of the chest: Neiguan(PC 6), Tanzhong(RN 17).

Hiccup: Gongsun(SP 4), Tiantu(RN 22).

Sudden aphonia: Tongli(HT 5), Lianquan(RN 23).

Convulsion: Hegu(LI 4), Yanglingquan(GB 34).

Loss of consciousness: Shuigou(DU 26), Yongquan(KI 1).

1.23 头痛
1.23 Headache

1.23.1 辨证
1.23.1 Differentiation

1.23.1.1 风邪外袭
1.23.1.1 Headache due to invasion of pathogenic wind into the meridians and collaterals

主要表现:恶风头痛,痛可及项背部。如头痛剧烈,刺痛,痛处不移,兼有脉弦,苔薄白者又称为"头风"。

Main manifestations: Headache occurs on exposure to wind, the pain may extend to the nape of the neck and back regions. If it is a violent, boring and fixed pain, accompanied by string-taut pulse and thin white tongue coating, shch a syndrome is also termed "head wind".

1.23.1.2 肝阳上亢

1.23.1.2 Headache due to upsurge of Liver-Yang

主要表现：头痛，眼花，双侧头痛剧烈，烦躁易怒，面赤口苦，脉弦数，舌红苔黄。

Main manifestations: Headache, blurred vision, severe pain on the bilateral sides of the head, irritability, hot temper, flushed face, bitter taste in the mouth, string-taut and rapid pulse, reddened tongue with yellow coating.

1.23.1.3 气血两虚

1.23.1.3 Headache due to deficiency of both Qi and blod

主要表现：头痛日久，头晕眼花，倦怠，面色无华，头痛得热则解，遇寒加剧，或遇劳累、情志不畅加重，舌淡苔薄白，脉细弱。

Main manifestations: Lingering headache, dizziness, blurred vision, lassitude, lustreless face, pain relieved by warmth and aggravated by cold, overstrain or mental stress, weak and thready pulse, pale tongue with thin and white coating.

临床上头痛辨证也要按头痛的位置及相应的经脉循行而定。颈项及枕部头痛属太阳经，前额及眉棱骨痛属阳明经，双侧及颞部痛属少阳经，以及巅顶痛属肝经、督脉。

Clinically varieties of headache should also differentiated according to the locality and the related meridians and collaterals. Pain in the occipital region and nape of the neck is related to the Bladder meridian of Foot-Taiyang, pain at the forehead and supraorbital region is related to the Stomach meridian of Foot-Yangming, pain in bilateral or unilateral temporal region is related to the Gallbladder meridian of Foot-Shaoyang, and that in the parietal region is related to the Liver meridian of Foot-Jueyin.

1.23.2 治疗
1.23.2 Treatment

1.23.2.1 风邪外袭
1.23.2.1 Headache due to invassion of pathogenic wind into meridians and collaterals

治疗原则:疏风解表,调理气血止头痛。局部和远端取穴相配合。施以泻法并留针。

处方:

枕部头痛:风池、昆仑、后溪;

前额痛:头维、印堂、上星、合谷、内庭;

颞侧痛:太阳、率谷、外关、足三里;

巅顶痛:百会、后溪、太冲、至阴。

上述穴位是依局部和远端取穴相配合的原则而定的。

枕部头痛取手足太阳经俞穴;

前额痛取手足阳明经俞穴;

颞侧痛取手足少阳经俞穴;

巅顶痛取手足太阳经、督脉及足厥阴肝经穴。

Principle of treatment: To dispel wind, remove obstruction in the meridians and collaterals, regulate the Qi and blood and relieve the pain by needling the local points and distal points along the related meridians. The reducing method with retention of needle is advisable.

Prescription:

Occiptal headache: Fengchi(GB 20), Kunlun(BL 60), Houxi(SI 3).

Frontal headache: Touwei(ST 8), Yintang (EX-HN 3), Shangxing (DU 23), Hegu(LI 4), Neiting(ST 44).

Temporal Headache: Taiyang (EX-HN 15), Shuaigu (GB 8). Waiguan(SJ 5), Zulinqu(ST 41).

Pauietal headache: Balhui(DU 20), Houxi(SI 3), Zhiyin(BL 67), Taichong(LR 3).

The above prescriptions are formulated by combining local points with distal points according to the location of headache and the affected meridian.

Occipital headache: points of the Taiyang meridians of Hand and Foot.

Frontal headache: points of the Yangming meridians of Hand and Foot.

Temporal headache: points of the Shaoyang meridians of Hand and Foot.

Parietal headache: points of the Taiyang meridians of Hand and Foot, those of the Jueyin meridian of Foot and those of Du meridian.

1.23.2.2 肝阳上亢
1.23.2.2 Headache due to upsurge of Liver-Yang

处方：风池、百会、悬颅、侠溪、行间。

施以泻法以平熄肝阳。

Prescription: Fengchi(GB 20), Baihui(DU 20), Xuanlu(GB 5), Xiaxi(GB 43), Xingjian(LR 2).

Needle with reducing method to pacify the Liver-Yang.

1.23.2.3 气血虚弱
1.23.2.3 Headache due to deficiency of both Qi and blood

处方：百会、气海、肝俞、脾俞、肾俞、足三里。

施以补法。

Prescription: Baihui (DU 20), Qihai (RN 6), Ganshu (BL 18), Pishu(BL 20), Shenshu(BL 23), Zusanli(ST 36).

Needle with reinforcing method.

1.24 三叉神经痛
1.24 Trigeminal Neuralgia

1.24.1 辨证
1.24.1 Differentiation

1.24.1.1 风寒外袭
1.24.1.1 Invasion by pathogenic wind and cold

主要表现:突发疼痛如电击,痛如刀割,烧灼感,不可忍,疼痛呈阵发性,一过性。每次发作持续数秒至数分钟,一日之中可发数次。同时可在眶上孔、眶下孔、颧骨出口处找到痛点,当按压这些痛点可诱发发作。疼痛经常伴有局部痉挛,流涕,流泪,流涎或伴见表证,脉来弦紧。

Main manifestations: Abrupt onset of pain occurs like an electric shock. The pain is cuting, boring and intolerable, but transient and proxysmal. Each attack lasts a few seconds or one to two minutes. It may recur several times a day. Tender points can be found on the supraobital foramen, infraorbital foramen, cheek foramen, lateral side of ala nasi, angle of the mouth, and nasolabial groove, where pressure induces the attack of pain. The pain is often accompanied by local spasm, running nose and lacrimation, salivation, or by symptoms of exterior syndrome with string-taut and tense pulse.

1.24.1.2 肝胃火盛

1.24.1.2 **Excesisve fire in the liver and stomach**

主要表现：三叉神经痛发作如前述，伴见烦躁易怒，口干便秘，舌苔黄干，脉弦数。

Main manifestations: The attack of pain as described above is accompnied by irritability, hot temper, thirst, constipation, yellow and dry tongue coating, and string-taut, rapid pulse.

1.24.1.3 **阴虚火旺**

1.24.1.3 **Deficiency of Yin and excessive fire**

主要表现：持续疼痛，消瘦，两颧潮红，腰酸倦怠，劳累后面疼加重，舌红少苔，脉细数。

Main manifestations: Insidious pain, emaciation, malar flush, sorness in the lumbar region, lassitude, pain aggravated by fatigue, thready and rapid pulse, reddened tongue with little coating.

1.24.2 治疗

1.24.2 Treatment

依据痛的部位及所影响到经脉局部取穴和远端配穴相结合。
处方：
眶上区痛：阳白、太阳、攒竹、外关；
上颌区痛：四白、颧骨、迎香、合谷；
下颌区痛：下关、颊车、大迎、合谷。
配穴：
风寒外袭：风池；
肝胃火盛：太冲、内庭；
阴虚火旺：照海、三阴交。

风寒外袭者施以泻法以祛散局部风寒之邪；肝胃实火者以泻法以清热泻火；至于阴虚火旺者，施以补法以滋阴降火。

To select the local points in combination with distal points according to the location of pain and the meridians affected.

Prescription:

Pain at supraorbital region: Xangbai (GB 14), Taiyang (EX-Hn 15), Zanzhu (BL 2), Waiguan (SJ 5).

Pain at maxillary region: Sibai (ST 2), Quanliao (SI 18), Yingxiang (LI 20), Hegu (LI 4).

Pain at mandibular region: Xiaguan (St 7), Jiache (ST 6), Daying (ST 5) Hegu (LI 4)).

Supplementary points:

Invasion by pathogenic wind and cold: Fengchi (GB 20).

Excessive fire in the liver and stomach: Taichong (LR 3) and Neiting (St 44).

Deficiency of Yin and excessive fire: Zhaohai (KI 6) and Sanyinjiao (SP 6)

For the invasion of pathogenic wind and cold, reducing method is used to promote the circulation of Qi and blood in the diseased area. For the excessive fire in the liver and stomach, reducing method is applied to bring down the fire. Reinforcing method is used in the type of deficiency of Yin and excessive fire to nourish the Yin and to dissipate the fire.

1.25 周围性面瘫
1.25 Peripheral Facial Paralysis

1.25.1 辨证
1.25.1 Differentiation

主要表现:起病突然,多于晨起发觉。患侧眼闭合不全,口角歪斜,流涎;不能皱额,不能皱眉、闭眼、鼓腮、露齿和吹口哨;甚者下颌痛,头痛,苔白,脉浮紧或浮缓。

Main manifestations: Sudden onset, usually right after waking up, incomplete closure of the eye in the affected side, drooping of the angle of the mouth, salivation and inability to frown, raise the eyebrow, close the eye, blow out the cheek, show the teeth or whistle, and in some cases pain in the mastoid region or headache, thin white tongue coating, superficial tense or superficial slow pulse.

1.25.2 治疗
1.25.2 Treatment

处方:翳风、阳白、太阳、颧髎、下关、地仓、颊车、合谷。
配穴:
皱额、皱眉困难:攒竹、丝竹空;
闭眼不全:攒竹、睛明、瞳子髎、鱼腰、丝竹空;
人中沟歪斜:人中;
露齿困难:巨髎;
耳鸣、耳聋:听会;

乳突压痛：完骨、外关。

针施以泻法。

病程长者在太阳、颊车、地仓、巨髎及下关穴施以温针或灸。

Prescription：Yifeng(SJ 17), Yangbai(GB 14), Taiyang(EX-HN 15), Quanliao (SI 18), Xiaguan(ST 7), Dicang(ST 4), Jiacahe(St 6), Hegu(LI 4).

Supplementary points：

Headache：Fengchi(GB20).

Difficulty in frowning and raising the eyebrow：Zhanzhu(BL 2), Sizhukong(SJ 23).

Incomplete closing of the eye：Zhanzhu(BL 2), Jingming(BL 1), Tongziliao(GB 1), Yuyao(EX-HN 4), Sizhukong(SJ 23).

Deviation of the philtrum：Renzhong(DU 26).

Inability to show the teeth：Juliao(ST 3).

Tinnitus and deafness：Tinghui(GB 2).

Tenderness at the mastoid region：Wangu(GB 12), Waiguan(SJ 5).

Needle all above points with reducing method.

In long-standing cases, the warming needle or moxibustion may be used to the points Taiyang(EX-Hn 15), Jiache (ST 6), Dicang(ST 4), Juliao(ST 3), and Xiaguan(ST 7).

1.26 胁痛
1.26 Pain in Hypochondriac Region

1.26.1 辨证
1.26.1 Differentiation

1.26.1.1 气滞
1.26.1.1 Stagnation of Qi

主要表现：胁肋胀痛，胸闷喜叹息，纳呆，口苦，苔薄白，脉弦。症状随情绪波动而变化。

Main manifestations: Distending pain in the costal and hypochondriac region, stuffing sensation in the chest, sighing, poor appetite, bitter taste in the mouth, thin white tongue coating, string-taut pulse. Severity of the symptoms varies with the changes of the emotional state.

1.26.1.2 血瘀
1.26.1.2 Stagnation of blood

主要表现：胁痛，疼痛固定如刺，夜间加剧，按之尤甚，舌质暗紫，脉沉涩。

Main manifestations: Fixed stabbing pain in the hypochondriac region, intensified by pressure and at night, dark pruplish tongue proper, deep and hesitant pulse.

1.26.1.3 肝阴不足
1.26.1.3 Deficiency of Liver Yin

主要表现：胁痛绵绵，口干，烦躁易怒，头晕眼花，舌红少苔，脉细弱而数。

Main manifestations: Dull pain lingering in the costal and hypochondriac region, dryness of the mouth, irritability, dizziness, blurring of vision, red tongue with little coating, weak, or rapid and thready pulse.

1.26.2 治疗
1.26.2 Treatment

1.26.2.1 气滞、血瘀
1.26.2.1 Stangnation of Qi and blood

处方:期门、支沟、阳陵泉。
气滞加:太冲、丘墟;
血瘀加:膈俞、肝俞。
针施以泻法。

Prescription: Qimen(LR 14), Zhigou(SJ 6), Yanglingquan(GB 34).

For stagnation of Qi, plus Taichong(LR 3) and Qiuxu (GB 40).
For stagnation of blood, plus Geshu(BL 17) and Ganshu(BL 18).
Needle all above points with reducing method.

1.26.2.2 肝阴不足
1.26.2.2 Deficiency of Liver Yin

处方:期门、肝俞、肾俞、足三里、三阴交、太冲。
针施以补泻并用。

Prescription: Qimen(LR 14), Ganshu(BL 18), Shenshu (BL 23), Zusanli(St 36), Sanyinjiao(SP 6), Taichong (LR 3).

Needle them with reinforcing methed.

1.27 腰痛
1.27 Low Back Pain

临床腰痛可由许多疾病引起,本节所论包括:寒湿外侵,肾气不足,外伤。

Clinically, low back pain can be found in various diseases. This section only deals with the following etiological factors: invasion of exogenous pathogenic cold and damp; deficiency of Qi of the kidney; and sprain or contusion.

1.27.1 辨证
1.27.1 Differentiation

1.27.1.1 寒湿外侵
1.27.1.1 Invasion of pathogenic cold and damp

主要表现:腰痛经常发生在居处寒湿环境之后,雨天加剧,腰背肌肉重着,仰俯不利,疼痛向臀部和下肢放射,患处寒冷,舌苔白腻,脉沉弱或沉迟。

Main manifestations: Low back pain usually occuring after exposure to cold and damp and aggravated on rainy days, heavy sensation and stiffness of the muscles in the dorsolumbar region, limitation of extension and flexion of the back, pain radiating downwards to the buttocks and lower limbs, cold feeling of the affected area, white and sticky tongue coating, deep and weak, or deep and slow pulse.

1.27.1.2 肾虚

1.27.1.2 **Kidney deficiency**

主要表现：腰痛迁延，起病缓慢，伴见腰膝酸软，劳累加剧，休息缓解。肾阳虚者可有下腹抽掣感，面色㿠白，肢冷，舌苔白，脉沉细或沉迟；肾阴虚者可有烦躁失眠，口咽干燥，面红，五心烦热，舌红少苔，脉细弱或细数。

Main manifestations: Insidious onset of protracted pain and soreness, accompanied by lassitude and weakness of the loins and knees, aggravated by fatigue and alleviated by bed rest. In case of deficiency of kidney Yang, cramp-like sensation in the lower abdomen, pallor, normal taste in the mouth, cold limbs, pale tongue, deep thready or deep slow pulse. In case of kidney Yin insufficiency, irritability, insomnia, dry mouth and throat, flushed face, feverish sensation in the chest, palms and soles, reddened tongue proper with scanty coating, thready weak or thready rapid pulse.

1.27.1.3 **外伤腰痛**

1.27.1.3 **Trauma**

主要表现：腰部外伤史，通常固定于腰部某一部位拘急疼痛，压之或运动时疼痛加剧，舌淡红或暗紫，脉弦涩。

Main manifestations: History of sprain of the lumbar region, rigidity and pain of the lower back which is generally fixed in a certain area, and is aggravated by pressure and by turning the body, pink or dark purplish tongue proper, string-taut hesitant pulse.

1.27.2 治疗

1.27.2 Treatment

塞湿外侵施以泻法并灸；肾虚者施以补法，阳虚可灸，外伤者施以泻法。

处方：肾俞、腰阳关、委中。
加减：
寒湿腰痛：大肠俞、关元俞；
肾阴虚者：志室、太溪；
肾阳虚者：关元、命门
外伤：人中、腰痛点、阿是穴。

Exogenous invasion by cold and dampness, punctured with reducing method and combining with moxibustion; Syndrome of kidney defieiency treated with reinforcing method, for kidney yang aeficiency could combine with moxibustion. For external injury treated with reducing mwthod.

Prescription: Shenshu (BL 23), Yaoyangguan (DU 3), Weizhong (BL 40).

Supplementary points:

Cold damp: Dachangshu (BL 25), Guanyuanshu (BL 26).

Deficiency of the kidney Yin: Zhishi (BL 52) and Taixi (KI 3).

Deficiency of the kidney Yang: Guanyuan (CV 4) and Mingmen (GV 4).

Traumatic injury: Renzhong (DU 26), Yaotongdian (EX-UE 7), and Ahshi point.

腰痛只是现代医学某个疾病的一个症状，如肾病、风湿病、类风湿、关节炎、脊柱增生、外伤及腰肌劳损。有时针灸只能作为一种辅助疗法。须积极治疗原发病。

Low back pain is only a symptom of some diseases such as renal diseases, rheumatism, rheumatoid arthritis, hyperplastic spondilitis, muscle strain or traumatic injury of the lumbar region in modern medicine. Sometimes acupuncture is only a supplementary method of treatment. The original disease should be treated actively.

1.28 痹证
1.28 Bi-syndrome

1.28.1 辨证
1.28.1 Differentiation

1.28.1.1 行痹
1.28.1.1 Wandering Bi

主要表现:关节游走疼痛,特别是在腕、肘、膝、踝关节;活动受限,恶寒发热,舌苔薄腻,脉浮紧或浮缓。

Main manifestations: Wandering pain in the joints, especially the wrists, elbows, knees and ankles; limitation of movement, chills and fever, thin and sticky tongue coating, superficial and tight or superficial and slow pulse.

1.28.1.2 痛痹
1.28.1.2 Painful Bi

主要表现:疼痛剧烈,得热则舒,遇寒痛甚,痛处固定,无红及热感,舌苔薄白,脉弦紧。

Main manifestations: Severe stabbing pain in the joints, alleviated by warmth and aggravated by cold, with fixed localization but no local redness and hotness, thin and white tongue coating, string-taut and tense pulse.

1.28.1.3 着痹
1.28.1.3 Fixd Bi

主要表现:肢体麻木重着,关节酸痛,阴雨天加剧,舌苔白腻,脉濡。

Main manifestations:Numbness and heavy sensation of the limbs, soreness and fixed pain of the joints, aggravated on cloudy and rainy days, white and sticky tongue coating and soft pulse.

1.28.2 治疗
1.28.2 Treatment

可选用阿是穴及阳经的远近端穴位,以祛风散寒除湿。行痹治以泻法,可运用皮内针。对于痛痹,应用灸法较好,同时配以深进针及长时间留针。疼痛剧烈可用皮内针及隔姜灸。着痹针灸并用,或用温针,或梅花针叩打及拔罐配合运用。

处方:

按区选穴:

肩关节痛:肩髃、肩髎、肩贞、膈俞;

肩胛痛:天宗、秉风、肩外俞、膏肓;

肘痛:曲池、尺泽、天井、外关、合谷;

腕痛:阳池、阳谷、阳溪、外关;

手指滞着:阳谷、合谷、后溪;

手指麻木疼痛:后溪、三间、八邪;

腰部疼痛:人中、肾俞、腰阳关;

髋关节痛:环跳、居髎、悬钟;

大腿疼痛:秩边、承扶、阳陵泉、阴陵泉;

小腿麻木疼痛:承山、飞扬;

踝关节痛:解溪、商丘、丘墟、昆仑、太溪;

足趾痛:公孙、束骨、八风;

背部疼痛:水沟、肾俞、腰阳关;

通身痛:后溪、申脉、大包、膈俞、肩髃、曲池、合谷、阳池、环跳、阳陵泉、悬钟、解溪。

配穴:

行痹、脉痹:膈俞、血海;

痛痹:肾俞、关元;

着痹:足三里、商丘;

Ahshi points together with the local and distal points along the Yang meridians supplying the diseased area are selected for the purpose of eliminating wind, cold and damp. Wandering Bi is mainly treated by the reducing method. Subcutaneous needles may also be applied. For painful Bi, it is better to use moxibustion, and apply needling as an adjuvant treatment with deep insertion and prolonged retaining of the needles. For severe pain, intradermal needles or indrect moxibustion with ginger may be used. Fixed Bi may also be treated by combined acupuncture and moxibustion, or together with warming needle, or tapping plus cupping.

Prescription:

Points along the affected regions are selected.

Pain in the shoulder joint: Jianyu (LI 15), Jianliao (SJ 14), Jianzhen(SJ 19), Naoshu(SI 10).

Pain in the scapula: Tianzong (SI 11), Bingfeng (SI 12), Jianwaishu(SI 14) and Gaohuang(BL 43).

Pain in the elbow: Quchi(LI 11), Chize (LU 5), Tianjing(SJ 10), Waiguan(SJ 5), Hegu(LI 4).

Pain in the wrist: Yangchi(SJ 4), Yangxi(LI 5), Yanggu(SI 5), Waiguan(SJ 5).

Stiffness of the fingers: Yanggu(SI 5), Hegu(LI 4), Houxi(SI 3).

Numbness and pain in the fingers: Houxi(SI 3), Sanjian(LI 3), Baxie(EX-UE 9)

Pain in the lumbar region: Renzhong (DU 26), Shenzhu (DU 12), Yaoyangguan (DU 3).

Pain in the hip joint: Huantiao (GB 30), Juliao (GB 29), Xuanzhong (GB 39).

Pian in the thigh region: Zhibian (BL 54), Chengfu (BL 36), Yanglingquan (GB 34).

Pain in the knee joint: Dubi (ST 35), Xiyan (EX-LE 5), Yanglingquan (GB 34), Yinlinquan (SP 9).

Numbness and pain in the leg: Chengshan (BL 57), Feiyang (BL 58).

Pain in the ankle: Jiexi (ST 41), Shangqiu (SP 5), Qiuxu (GB 40), Kunlun (BL 60), Taixi (KI 3).

Numbenss and Pain in the toes: Gongsun (SP 4), Shugu (BL 65), Bafeng (EX-LE 10).

Pain in the back: Shuigou (DU 26), Shenzhu (DU 12), Yaoyangguan (DU 3).

General pain: Houxi (SI 3), Shenmai (BL 62), Dabao (SP 21), Geshu (BL 17), Jianyu (LI 15), Quchi (LI 11), Hegu (LI 4), Yangchi (SJ 4), Huantiao (GB 30), Yanglingquan (GB 34), Xuanzhong (GB 39), Jiexi (ST 41).

Supplementary points:

Wandering Bi, vessel Bi: Geshu (BL 17), Xuehai (SP 10); Painful Bi: Shenshu (BL 23), Guanyuan (RN 4); Fixed Bi: Zusanli (St 36), Shanqiu (SP 5).

1.29 痿证
1.29 Wei-Syndrome

痿证是以肌肉痿缩或痿软及运动障碍为特征的疾病。

The Wei syndrome is characterized by flaccidity or atrophy of the limbs with motor impairment.

1.29.1 辨证
1.29.1 Differentiation

1.29.1.1 肺热
1.29.1.1 Heat in the lung

主要表现：下肢肌肉痿软，运动受限，伴见发热，咳嗽，易怒，口渴，尿黄短，舌红苔黄，脉细数或滑数。

Main manifestations: Muscular flaccidity of the lower limbs with motor impairment, accompanied by fever, cough, irritability, thirst, scanty and brownish urine, reddened tongue with yellow coating, thready and rapid or rolling and rapid pulse.

1.29.1.2 湿热证
1.29.1.2 Damp heat

主要表现：小腿痿软微肿，触之微热，全身重着，胸闷脘痞，尿黄短，尿时疼痛，舌苔黄腻，脉濡数。

Main manifestations: Flaccid or slight swollen legs, a little hot sensation on touch, general heaviness, sensation of fullness in the chest and epigastric region, painful urination, hot and brownish urine, yellow sticky tongue coating, soft and rapid pulse.

1.29.1.3 肝肾阴虚
1.29.1.3 Deficiency of Yin of the liver and kidney

主要表现:下肢痿软,运动受限,腰部酸软无力,遗精,滑精,带下,头晕眼花,舌质红,脉细数。

Main manifestations: Muscular flaccidity of the lower limbs with motor impairment, combined with sorness and weakness of the lumbar region, seminal emission, prospermia, dizziness, blurring of vision, reddened tongue, thready and rapid pulse.

1.29.1.4 外伤
1.29.1.4 Trauma

主要表现:外伤之后,肢体痿瘫,或伴见二便失禁,脉涩,淡红或暗紫舌,苔薄或薄白。

Main manifestations: History of trauma, flaccid paralytic limbs, may be accompanied with incontinence of urine and feces, relaxed or hesitant pulse, pink or dark purplish tongue or thin or thin white coating.

1.29.2 治疗
1.29.2 Treatment

主要选取阳明经穴以疏通气血,滋润筋骨。如果热邪或湿热之邪在肺是主要病因,应以泻法清热;肝肾阴虚,施以补法;对外伤者以平补平泻法针患侧。

处方:

上肢:肩髃、曲池、合谷、外关;

下肢:髀关、环跳、血海、梁丘、足三里、阳陵泉、解溪、悬钟;

配穴:

肺热:尺泽、肺俞;

湿热:脾俞、阴陵泉;

肝肾阴虚：膈俞、肾俞；

外伤：相应于受损脊柱处的华佗夹脊；

大便失禁：大肠俞、次髎。

Main points are selected from the Yangming Meridians to promote circulation of Qi in the meridians, and to nourish the tendons and bones. If heat or damp heat in the lung is the main etiological factor, the reducing method should be used to dissipate heat. In case of deficiency of Yin in the liver and kidney, the reinforcing method should be employed. For trauma, puncture the points on the affected side with even method.

Prescription:

Upper limb: Jianyu(LI 15), Quchi(LI 11), Hegu(LI 4), Waiguan (SJ 5).

Lower limb: Biguan(ST 31), Huantiao(GB 30), Xuehai(SP 10), Liangqiu(ST 34), Zusanli(ST 36), Yanglingquan(GB 34), Jiexi(ST 41), Xuanzhong(GB 39).

Supplementary Points:

For the heat in the lung: Chize (LI 5), Feishu(BL 13).

For damp heat: Pishu(BL 20), Yinlingquan(SP 9).

Deficiency of Yin in the liver and kidney: Ganshu (BL 18) and Shenshu(BL 23).

For trauma: Huantuojiaji at the corresponding level of spinal injury.

Incontinence of feces: Dachangshu(BL 25), Ciliao(BL 32).

该证见于急性脊髓炎、进行性肌萎缩、重症肌无力、多发性神经炎、小儿麻痹后遗症、周期性麻痹、癔病之瘫痪、外伤性瘫痪等。

The syndrome is seen in acute myelitis, progressive myatrophy, myasthenia gravis, multiple neuritis, sequellae of poliomyelitis, periodic paralysis, hysterical paralysis, traumatic paraplegia, etc. in modern medicine.

第二章 妇儿科病症
CHAPTER TWO GYNECOLOGICAL AND PEDIATRIC DISEASES

2.1 月经不调
2.1 Irregular Menstruation

2.1.1 辨证
2.1.1 Differentiation

2.1.1.1 **月经先期**
2.1.1.1 **Antedated menstruation**

2.1.1.1.1 血热型
2.1.1.1.1 Heat in blood

主要表现:月经周期缩短,经血深红而粘稠,量多,胸闷烦躁,尿赤,舌红苔黄,脉数有力。

Main manifestations: Shortened cycle, dark red and thick blood flow in large quantities, restlessness, fullness in the chest, brown urine, reddened tongue with yellow coating, rapid and forceful pulse.

2.1.1.1.2 气虚型
2.1.1.1.2 Qi deficiency

主要表现:月经量多,色淡,周期缩短,疲乏心悸气短,下腹空而重着感,舌淡苔薄,脉弱。

Main manifestations: Profuse, thin and light red menses in shortened cycle, lassitude, palpitation, shortness of breath, subjective empty and heavy sensation in the lower abdomen, pale tongue with thin coating, weak pulse.

2.1.1.2 月经后期
2.1.1.2 Postdated menstruation:
2.1.1.2.1 血虚型
2.1.1.2.1 Blood deficiency

主要表现:月经周期延迟,月经量少色淡,下腹空痛,消瘦,面色萎黄,肌肤不荣,头晕眼花,心悸失眠,舌淡红少苔,脉细弱。

Main manifestations: Scanty and pink menses in delayed cycle, empty and painful feeling in the lower abdomen, emaciation, sallow complexion, lusterless skin, dizziness and blurred vision, palpitation and insomnia, pink tongue with little coating, weak and thready pulse.

2.1.1.2.2 血寒型
2.1.1.2.2 Cold in the blood

主要表现:月经周期推迟,量少色暗,下腹挚痛,得温稍减,肢冷,舌苔薄白,脉沉迟。

Main manifestations: Scanty and dark-coloured menses in delayed cycle, colic pain in the lower abdomen, slightly alleviated by warmth, cold limbs, thin and white tongue, deep and slow pulse.

2.1.1.2.3 气滞型
2.1.1.2.3 Qi stagnation

主要表现:月经周期推迟,量少色暗红,下腹胀痛,情绪抑郁,胸闷,呃逆,胸胁及乳房发胀,苔薄白,脉弦。

Main manifdstations: Scanty and dark red menses in delayed cycle, distending pain in the lower abdomen, mental depression, stuffy chest alleviated by belching, distension in the hypochondriac region and breast, thin, white tongue coating and string—taut pulse.

2.1.1.3 月经先后不定期
2.1.1.3 Irregular menstrual cycles

2.1.1.3.1 肝气郁结
2.1.1.3.1 Qi stagnation in the liver

主要表现:月经周期及经血量变化不定,月经血粘稠,色紫暗,排出困难,胸胁两乳发胀,下腹胀痛,精神抑郁,常叹息,舌苔白,脉弦。

Main manifestations: Alteration of menstrual cycles and quantity of blood flow, thick, sticky, and purple colored menses difficult to flow, distension in the hypochondriac region and breast, distending pain in the lower abdomen, mental depression, frequent sighing, thin white tongue coating and string—taut pulse.

2.1.1.3.2 肾虚
2.1.1.3.2 Kidney deficiency

主要表现:月经先后不定,量少色淡,头晕耳鸣,腰膝酸痛而软,夜尿频繁,便溏,舌淡苔薄,脉沉弱。

Main manifestations: Scanty, pink blood flow in irregular cycles, dizziness and tinnitus, weak and aching of the lower back and kness, frequent night urination, loose stools, pale tongue with thin coating, deep and weak pulse.

2.1.2 治疗
2.1.2 Treatment

2.1.2.1 月经先期

2.1.2.1 Antedated menstruation

2.1.2.1.1 血热
2.1.2.1.1 Heat in the blood

处方:曲池、中极、血海、水泉。

配穴:

肝郁化火:行间;

阴虚内热:然谷;

以泻法清热凉血,调整冲任。

Prescription: Quchi(LI 11), Zhongji(RN 3), Xuehai(SP 10), Shuiquan(KI 5).

Supplementary points:

Liver Qi transforming into fire: Xingjian(LR 2).

Yin deficiency with internal heat: Rangu(KI 2).

Acupuncture with the reducing method is applied to regulate the Chong and Ren Meridans, and clear off heat from blood.

2.1.2.1.2 气虚
2.1.2.1.2 Qi deficiency

处方:气海、三阴交、中脘、足三里。

施以补法。

Prescription: Qihai(RN 6), Sanyinjiao(SP 6), Zhongwan(RN 12), Zusanli(ST 36).

Acupuncture is applied with reinforcing method.

2.1.2.2 月经后期
2.1.2.2 Postdated menstruation

2.1.2.2.1 血虚及血寒
2.1.2.2.1 Blood deficiency and cold in the blood

处方:关元、气海、三阴交。

配穴:

头晕眼花:百会;心悸失眠:神门。

血虚者施以补法以补气生血。血寒者施以平补平泻,或灸以温经散寒。

Prescription: Guanyuan(RN 4), Qihai(RN 6), Sanyinjiao(SP 6).

Supplementary points:

Dizziness and blurred vision: Baihui(DU 20); Palpitation and insomnia:

Shenmen(HT 7).

In case of blood deficiency, acupunture is applied with the reinforcing method to replenish Qi and nourish blood. Moxibustion is also advisable. In case of cold in the blood, acupuncture is given with the even method. Strong stimulation of moxibustion is used to warm up the meridians and disperse cold.

2.1.2.2.2 气滞

2.1.2.2.2 Qi stagnation

处方:天枢、气穴、地机、太冲。

配穴:

胸闷:内关;胸乳胀:期门。

施以泻法。

Prescription: Tianshu(ST 25), Qixue(KI 13), Diji(ST 8), Taichong(LR 3).

Supplementary points:

Fullness of the chest: Neiguan(PC 4).

Distension in the hypochondriac region and breast: Qimen(LR 14).

Needle all above points with reducing method.

2.1.2.3 月经先后不定期

2.1.2.3 Irregular menstrual cycles

2.1.2.3.1 肝气郁结

2.1.2.3.1 Qi stagnation in the liver

处方：气海、四满、间使、蠡沟。

胸乳胀加膻中穴；情志抑郁加神门、太冲。

施以平补平泻法。

Prescription: Qihai(RN 6), Siman(KI 14), Jianshi(PC 5), Ligou(LR 5).

Supplementary points:

Distension in the hypochondriac region and breast: Tanzhong(RN 17), Qimen(LR 14).

Mental depression: Shenmen(HT 7), Taichong(LR 3).

Acupuncture is given with even method.

2.1.2.3.2 肾虚

2.1.2.3.2 Kidney deficiency

处方：关元、肾俞、交信。

腰膝酸软：腰眼、阴谷；头晕眼花：百会、太溪。

施以补法并灸。

Prescription: Guanyuan(RN 4), Shenshu(BL 23), Jiaoxin(KI 8).

Supplementary points:

Sore and weak low back and kness: Yaoyan(EX-B 7), Yingu(KI 10).

Dizziness and tinnitus: Baihui(DU 20), Taixi(KI 3).

Acupuncture is given with reinforcing method. Apply moxibustion.

该病包括垂体前叶功能失调或卵巢功能失调而引起的月经周期不规则。

This disorder includes the irregular menorrhea resulted form dysfunction of antehypophysis or from ovarian dysfunction.

2.2 痛经
2.2 Dysmenorrhea

2.2.1 辨证
2.2.1 Differentiation

2.2.1.1 实证
2.2.1.1 Excess syndrome

主要表现：下腹疼痛，通常起於月经期前，月经量少色暗紫挟有血块，下腹胀痛，血块排出痛减，胸乳作胀，舌暗紫或有瘀斑，脉沉弦；下腹泛痛连及腰背，月经量少色深红挟血块，苔白腻，脉沉弦。

Main manifestations: Pain in the lower abdomen, usually starting before menstruation, retarded, scanty and dark purple menses with clots, distending pain in the lower abdomen, alleviated by passing out the clots, distension in the hypochondriac region and breast, purplish tongue with purple spots on its edge, deep and string—taut pulse; pain and cold feeling in the lower abdomen referring to the waist and back, alleviated by warmth, scanty dark red menses with clots, sticky and white tongue coating, deep string—taut pulse.

2.2.1.2 虚证
2.2.1.2 Deficiency syndrome

主要表现：月经末期腹痛隐隐，得温或按压稍减，月经量少色淡,脉细弱,伴见恶寒肢冷,面色㿠白,心悸,头晕。

Main manifestations: Dull pain appearing by the end of or after menstruation, alleviated by warmth and pressure, pink, scanty and thin menses, thready and weak pulse accompanied by intolerance to cold, cold extremities, pale complexion, palpitation and dizziness.

2.2.2 治疗
2.2.2 Treatment

2.2.2.1 实证
2.2.2.1 Excess syndrome

处方:中极、次髎、合谷、血海、地机、太冲。针灸并用。
下腹胀痛加四满、水道;下腹冷痛加归来、大巨。

Prescription: Zhongji(RN 3), Ciliao(BL 32), Hegu(LI 4), Xuehai(SP 10), Diji(SP 8), Taichong(LR 3). Both acupuncture and moxibustion are used in case of cold syndrome.

Supplementary points:

Distending pain in the lower abdomen: Siman(KI 14), Shuidao(ST 28).

Pain with cold feeling in the lower abdomen: Guilai(ST 29), Daju(ST 27).

2.2.2.2 虚证
2.2.2.2 Deficiency syndrome

处方:关元、脾俞、肾俞、足三里、三阴交。
施以补法及灸法以调气血,温养冲任。

Prescription: Guanyuan(RN 4), Pishu(BL 20), Shenshu(BL 23), Zusanli(ST 36), Sanyinjiao(SP 6).

Acupuncture is given with the reinforcing method and moxibustion

173

to regualte the Qi and blood, warm up and nourish the Chong and Ren meridians.

2.3 闭经
2.3 Amenorrhea

2.3.1 辨证
2.3.1 Differentiation

2.3.1.1 血瘀
2.3.1.1 Blood stagnation

主要表现:月经数月不来,下腹胀痛拒按,下腹硬块,胸胁胀满,舌质暗紫边有瘀点,脉沉弦。

Main manifesttations: Absence of menses for months, lower abdominal distending pain aggravated by pressure, hard mass in lower abdomen, distension and fullness in the chest and hypochondriac region, dark purple tongue with purplish spots on its borders, deep string—taut pulse.

2.3.1.2 血虚
2.3.1.2 Blood depletion

主要表现:月经延迟,渐至经少闭经,久则面色萎黄,倦怠头晕昏眩,纳呆便溏,皮肤干燥,舌淡苔白,脉迟弱,全属气血不足之象;头晕耳鸣,腰膝酸软,口干,五心烦热,潮热盗汗,舌淡少苔,脉弦细,此则为精血不足之征。

Main manifestations: Delayed menstrual cycle, gradual decrease of menses and amenorrhea, sallow complexion in prolonged cases, lassitude, vertigo and dizziness, poor appetite, loose stools, dry skin, pale tongue with white coating, slow weak pulse, all of which are signs of deficiency of Qi and blood; dizziness and tinnitus, sore and weak low back and knees, dry mouth and throat, hot sensation in the palms, soles and epigastrium, afternoon fever and night sweating, pale tongue with little coating, string—taut and thready pulse, all of which are signs of deficiency of essence and blood.

2.3.2 治疗
2.3.2 Treatment

2.3.2.1 血瘀
2.3.2.1 Blood stagnation

处方:中极、归来、血海、太冲、合谷、三阴交。

下腹疼痛硬块且拒按者加四满穴。施以泻法以调通气血,祛瘀。

Prescription: Zhongji(RN 3), Guilai(ST 29), Xuehai(SP 10), Taichong(LR 3), Hegu(LI 4), Sanyinjiao(SP 6).

Pain in the lower abdomen with hard mass aggravated by pressure plus: Siman(KI 14).

Acupuncture with reducing method is used to remove the stagnation and regulate the circulation of Qi, and blood in the meridians.

2.3.2.2 血虚
2.3.2.2 Blood depletion

处方:关元、肝俞、脾俞、肾俞、足三里、三阴交。

施以针之补法,有时加灸以养血通经。

Prescription: Guanyuan(RN 4), Ganshu(BL 18), Pishu(BL 20), Shenshu(BL 23), Zusanli(ST 36), Sanyinjiao(SP 6).

Needle with reinforcing method. Moxibustion is applied sometimes to tonify blood and restore menses.

2.4 崩漏
2.4 Uterine Bleeding

2.4.1 辨证
2.4.1 Differentiation

2.4.1.1 实热
2.4.1.1 Excessive heat

主要表现:突然大量或长期持续阴道流血,色深红,烦躁失眠,头晕,舌红,苔黄脉数。

Main manifestation: Sudden onset of profuse or prolonged continuous vaginal bleeding in deep red colour, fidgets, insomnia, dizziness, red tongue with yellow coating, rapid pulse.

2.4.1.2 气虚
2.4.1.2 Qi deficiency

主要表现:突然大量出血或长期小量流血,色淡质稀,倦怠,气短懒言,纳呆便溏,舌质淡,脉细弱。

Main manifestations: Sudden profuse bleeding or continuous scanty bleeding marked by pink and thin blood, lasstidue, shortness of breath, apathy, anorexia, loose stools, pale tongue, thready weak pulse.

2.4.2 治疗
2.4.2 Treatment

2.4.2.1 实热
2.4.2.1 Excessive heat
处方：中极、血海、隐白、曲泉。
配穴：
内热证：曲池；心火旺盛：少府；肝火旺盛：太冲。
施以泻法清热止血。

Prescription：Zhongji(RN 3), Xuehai(SP 10), Yinbai(SP 1), Ququan(LR 8).

Supplementary points：

Affection of internal heat：Quchi(LI 11). Excessive heart fire：Shaofu(HT 8). Excessive liver fire：Taichong(LR 3). Acupuncture with reducing method is used to clear off heat and stop bleeding.

2.4.2.2 气虚
2.4.2.2 Qi deficiency
处方：百会、关元、足三里、三阴交、隐白、阳池。
配穴：脾气虚弱，纳呆便溏：脾俞、胃俞。
施以补法及灸法以补气摄血。

Prescription：Baihui(DU 20), Guanyuan(RN 4), Zusanli(ST 36), Sanyinjiao(SP 6), Yinbai(SP 1), Yangchi(SJ 14).

Supplementary points：

Spleen Qi deficiency manifested by anorexia and loose stools：Pishu(BL 20), Weishu(BL 21).

Acupuncture with reinforcing method and moxibustion are employed to promote the restricting function of Qi.

2.5 带下病
2.5 Morbid leukorrhea

2.5.1 辨证
2.5.1 Differentiation

2.5.1.1 脾虚
2.5.1.1 Deficiency in the spleen

主要表现:白带量多粘稠,色白或稍黄而无臭味,面色苍白或萎黄,疲乏,纳呆便溏,下肢水肿,舌淡苔白腻,脉迟而弱。

Main manifestations: Profuse thick, white or light yellowish vaginal discharge without smell, pale or sallow complexion, lassitude, poor appetite and loose stools, edema in the lower limbs, pale tongue with white sticky coating, slow weak pulse.

2.5.1.2 肾虚
2.5.1.2 Deficiency in the Kidney

主要表现:白带清稀量多,绵绵不绝,腰背极度酸软,下腹冷,尿多清长,大便稀溏,舌淡苔薄,脉沉。

Main manifestations: Profue and continuous discharge of thin and clear white, severe soreness of the low back, cold sensation in the lower abdomen, frequent and excessive urine, loose stools, pale tongue with thin coating, and deep pulse.

2.5.1.3 湿热
2.5.1.3 Damp heat

主要表现:白带量多,黄稠而粘,有腥臭味,外阴搔痒,大便干结,尿黄,脉濡数,苔黄腻;或白带赤黄相间,口干咽干,烦热躁扰,心悸失眠,舌苔黄,脉弦数。

Main manifestations: Sticky, viscous and stinking yellow leukorrhea in large quantity, itching in the vulva, dry stool, scanty and yellow urine, soft and rapid pulse, sticky yellow coating, or leukorrhea in reddish yellow colour, bitter taste in the mouth, dry throat, irritability with a feverish sensation, palpitation, insomnia, yellow coating, string-taut and rapid pulse.

2.5.2 治疗
2.5.2 Treatment

2.5.2.1 脾虚
2.5.2.1 Deficiency in the spleen

处方:带脉、气海、白环俞、阴陵泉、足三里。

施以补法和灸法以健脾祛湿,调冲摄带。

Prescription: Daimai(BL 26), Qihai(RN 6), Baihuanshu(BL 30), Yinlingquan(SP 9), Zusanli(ST 36).

Acupuncture with the reinforcing mehtod and moxibustion is used to build up the spleen and remove damp, regulate Ren meridian and stabilize Dai meridian.

2.5.2.2 肾虚
2.5.2.2 Deficiency in the Kidney

处方:肾俞、关元、大赫、带脉、复溜。

施以补法及灸法以强肾气固冲任。

Prescription: Shenshu(BL 23), Guanyuan(RN 4), Dahe(KI 12), Daimai(BL 26) Fuliu(KI 7).

Acupuncture with the reinforcing method and moxibution are used to promote Yang Qi, tonify the kidney and stablize the Ren and Dai meridians.

2.5.2.3 湿热
2.5.2.3 Damp heat

处方：中极、次髎、三阴交、太冲。

外阴搔痒加蠡沟；赤带加曲池、血海；实热证加曲池。

施以泻法以清热祛湿，调摄任带二脉。

Prescription: Zhongji(RN 3), Ciliao(BL 32), Sanyinjiao(SP 6), Taichong(LR 3).

Supplementary points: Itching in the vulva: Ligou(LR 5). Reddish leukorrhea: Quchi(LI 11). Xuehai(SP 10) Excessive heat: Quchi (LI 11).

Acupuncture with the reducing method is employed to clear off heat, remove damp, adjust the Ren meridian and stabilize Dai meridian.

2.6 妊娠呕吐
2.6 Morning sickness

2.6.1 辨证
2.6.1 Differentiation

2.6.1.1 脾胃虚弱
2.6.1.1 Deficiency in the spleen and stomach

主要表现：进食之后立即恶心或呕吐未消化之食物，或吐水，胸中胀满，倦怠思睡，舌淡苔白，妊娠早期脉滑而无力。

Main manifestations: Nausea and vomiting of liquid or indigested food immediately after meals, fullness and distending feeling in the chest, lassitude and sleepiness, pale tongue with white coating, slippery and weak pulse during the early stage of pregnancy.

2.6.1.2 肝胃不和

2.6.1.2 Disharmony between the Liver and Stomach

主要表现:呕吐酸水或苦水,胁痛脘胀,呃逆频频,善喜叹息,精神抑郁,头晕、双眼发胀,舌苔黄,妊娠早期脉来弦滑。

Main manifestations: Vomiting of bitter or sour liquid, epigastric fullness and hyperchondriac pain, frequent belching and sighing, mental depression, dizziness and eye distension, yellowish tongue coating and string—taut slippery pulse in the early stage of gestation.

2.6.2 治疗

2.6.2 Treatment

2.6.2.1 脾胃虚弱

2.6.2.1 Deficiency in the spleen and stomach

处方:中脘、上脘、内关、足三里、公孙。

施以平补平泻法以健脾和胃,降逆止呕。

Prescription: Zhongwan(RN 12), Shangwan(RN 13), Neiguan(PC 6), Zusanli(ST 36), Gongsun(SP 4).

Acupuncture with even method is applied to build up the spleen, harmonize the stomach and check the adversive flowing of Qi so as to stop vomiting.

2.6.2.2 肝胃不和

2.6.2.2 Disharmony between the liver and stomach

处方:膻中、中脘、内关、足三里、太冲。

Prescription: Tanzhong(RN 17), Zhongwan(RN 12), Neiguan (PC 6), Zusanli(ST 36), Taichong(LR 3).

早期妊娠不可在许多穴位上施针,也不宜以强制激,以免损伤胎气。应让病人卧床休息,避免生冷、油腻食品。为使胃气渐复可让病人少吃多餐。

Acupuncture should not be applied to many points, nor with strong stimulation when the fetus is still young in the early stage of gestation, lest the fetal Qi should be affected. It is appropriate to keep the patient in bed and away from raw, cold or greasy food. In the hope of adjusting and replenishing the stomach Qi, multiple meals with a little intake of food is advisable.

2.7 乳汁不足
2.7 Insufficient Lactation

2.7.1 辨证
2.7.1 Differentiation

2.7.1.1 气血不足
2.7.1.1 Deficiency of Qi and blood

主要表现:产后乳少或缺乳,或哺乳期乳汁不足,乳房无胀痛,面色苍白,皮肤无光泽,心悸气短,纳呆便溏,舌淡少苔,脉来细弱。

Main manifestations: Insuffcient secretion of milk after delivery or even absence of milk , or decreasing secretion during lactation period, no distending pain in the breast, pale complexion, dry skin, palpitation, lassitude, poor appetite, loose stools, pale tongue with little coating, weak and thready pulse.

2.7.1.2 肝气郁结
2.7.1.2 Liver Qi stagnation

主要表现：产后无乳，乳房胀痛，精神抑郁，胸闷胁痛，胃脘胀满，纳呆，舌淡红，苔薄白，脉弦。

Main manifestations: Absence of milk secretion after delivery, distending pain in breast, mental depression, chest distress and hypochondriac pain, epigastric distension, loss of appetite, pink tongue with thin coating, string—taut pulse.

2.7.2 治疗
2.7.2 Treatment

主要选取足阳明经穴。气血不足患者施以补法及灸法以补益气血，促进乳汁分泌；肝气郁结者，施以泻法或平补平泻法，或适当辅以灸法以疏肝解郁、疏通气血，促进排乳。

处方：乳根、膻中、少泽。

气血不足辅以脾俞、足三里、三阴交；肝气郁结者加上期门、内关、太冲。

治疗期间产妇应加强营养，多进汤水及采用正确喂养方法。

Mainly select the points from the Foot — Yangming Meridian. Acupucture is given with reinforcing method and moxibustion in case of deficiency of Qi and blood to tonify the Qi and blood in order to promote lactic secretion. Acupuncture with either reducing or even method or with appropriate moxibustion in case of liver Qi stagnation is to remove the stagnation of liver Qi, to promote secretion of milk.

Prescription: Rugen(ST 28), Tanzhong(RN 17), Shaoze(SI 1).

Supplementary points:

Deficiency of Qi and blood: Pishu(BL 20), Zusanli(ST 36), Sanyinjiao(SP 6).

Liver Qi stagnation: Qimen(LR 14), Neiguan(PC 6), Taichong (LR 3).

When receiving acupuncture for insufficient lactation, it is very important that the mother have nutrient diet, take plenty of soup , and apply correct nursing method.

2.8 婴儿腹泻
2.8 Infantile Diarrhoea

2.8.1 辨证
2.8.1 Differentiation

主要表现：肠鸣腹胀，频繁阵发腹痛，腹痛多在肠蠕动之后，排便后腹痛缓解。

一日可有数次酸腐便。腹泻由于喂养过度引起者表现为粪中挟有不消化之乳食，嗳气频频，纳呆，舌苔腻。由於湿热引起者，大便稀黄而臭，腹痛，发热口渴，肛门均热感，小便短赤，舌苔黄腻。

Main manifestatios: Abdominal distension is accompanied by borborygmi and frequent fits of pain. The fit of pain is followed by bowel movements, and the pain will be relieved after .

There are several times of defecation a day with sour and putrid feces. The diarrhoea caused by overfeeding is marked by presence of undigested milk and food in the discharge, frequent eructation, anorexia, sticky tongue coating. In diarrhoea caused by damp heat ,there are loose stools with yellow colour and offensive smell, abdominal pain, fever and thirst, burning sensation at the anus, scanty and dark urine, yellow and sticky tongue coating.

2.8.2 治疗

2.8.2 Treatmeant

在足阳明胃经穴位上施以针刺以调整脾胃功能,清热利湿止泻。

处方:天枢、上巨墟、四缝。

配穴:湿热泻曲池、合谷、阴陵泉;由于喂养过度者配以建里,气海穴。

严重腹泻会导致阴阳受损,或气随液脱的重症,需加注意。治疗期间需控制饮食,以少量清淡饮食为佳。

Points of Foot Yangming meridian are mainly recommended to adjust the spleen and stomach, eliminate damp heat and stop diarrhoea.

prescription: Tianshu(ST 25), Shangjuxu(ST 37), Sifeng(EX-UE 10).

Supplementary points:

Diarrhoea due to overfeeding: Jianli(RN 11), Qihai(RN 6).

Attention should be paid to severe diarrhoea which may lead to the critical condition of the damage of both Yin and Yang, collapse of Qi and exhaustion of Yin.

During the treatment, the patient should take a restricted and a light diet of small quantity.

2.9 小儿疳积
2.9 Infantile Malnutrition

2.9.1 辨证
2.9.1 differentiation

主要表现:逐渐起病,午后潮热或低热,口干腹胀,腹泻大便恶臭,尿如米泔水,烦躁啼哭,食欲不佳。由于积滞内停,肚大脐突,面色萎黄,形体消瘦,肌肤甲错,头发稀疏,舌苔腐腻,或舌苔全剥,脉弱。上述诸症与脾胃虚弱有关。

Main manifestations: Gradual onset of slight fever or tidal fever in the afternoon, dryness of the mouth, abdominal distension, diarrhoea with offensive odour, rice—water like urine, crying with irritability, and anorexia. Then, distended belly with protruding umbilicus due to internal stagnation, sallow complexion, emaciation, scaly and dry skin, sparse hair, dirty and sticky coating of the tongue, or complete loss of coating, and weak pulse. The above symptoms are related to deficiency of the spleen and stomach.

2.9.2 治疗
2.9.2 Treatment

选取足阳明经脉俞穴及背俞穴为主以健脾消积,施以毫针浅刺,不留针。

处方:下脘、胃俞、脾俞、足三里、四缝、太白。百虫窝(经外奇穴)常用於"疳虫"内积。

Points of foot Taiying and foot Yangming meridians are selected to reinforce the spleen and remove the stagnation. Superficial pricking with filiform needles is applied and the needles are not retained.

Prescription: Xiawan(RN 10), Weishu(BL 21), Pishu(BL 20), Zusanli(ST 36), Sifeng(EX—UE 10), Taibai(SP 3).

Baichongwo(EX—LE 3) is used as a supplementary point for parasitosis.

第三章 眼、耳、鼻、喉及外科诸证
CHAPTER THREE
EXTERNAL DISEASES AND DISEASES OF EYES, EARS, NOSE AND THROAT

3.1 荨麻疹
3.1 Urticaria

3.1.1 辨证
3.1.1 Differentiation

突然起病,风团搔痒,形态各异,此起彼伏,或疹块突起,或连成片。可因气候变化而加剧或渐减。急性患者消退迅速,按临床症状可分为如下几型。

Abrupt onset with itching wheals of various size or with pimples rising one after another. It might be aggravated or lessened by the changing of weather. Acute conditions subside quickly. It is divided into the following types according to clinical symptoms.

3.1.1.1 风热型
3.1.1.1 wind heat

主要表现:红色风团,皮肤奇痒,脉浮数。

Main manifestations: Red rashes with severe itching, superficial and rapid pulse.

3.1.1.2 风湿型
3.1.1.2 Wind damp
主要表现:风团色淡或色白伴有肢体困重,舌苔白腻,脉浮缓。

Main manifestations: White or pink rashes accompanied by heaviness of the body, superficial and slow pulse, white and sticky tongue coating.

3.1.1.3 肠胃积热
3.1.1.3 Accumulation of heat in the stomach and intestines
主要表现:风团块,伴有脘腹疼痛,便秘或腹泻,苔薄黄,脉数。

Main manifestations: Red rashes complicated by abdominal or epigastric pain, constipation or diarrhoea, thin yellow tongue coating and rapid pulse.

3.1.2 治疗
3.1.2 Treatment

施以泻法以祛风湿、清血热,主要选取脾与大肠经俞穴。局部梅花针叩打亦可。

处方:曲池、合谷、委中、血海、三阴交。

风热者加大椎;风湿者加阴陵泉;胃肠积热同时针天枢、足三里。

The reducing method is used to disperse wind damp and eliminate heat in the blood. Points of the spleen adn large intestine meridians are selected as the principal points. Tapping on the affected area with a "plum—blossom" needle is advisable.

Prescription: Quchi(LI 11), Hegu(Li 4), Weizhong(BL 40), Xuehai(SP 10), Sanyinjiao(SP 6).

Supplementary points:

Wind heat: Dazhui(DU 14)

Wind damp: Yinlingquan(SP 9)

Accumulation of heat in the stomach and intestines: Tianshu(ST 25), Zusanli(ST 36).

3.2 带状疱疹
3.2 Herpes Zoster

3.2.1 辨证
3.2.1 Differentiation

带状疱疹多见于腰背部,呈带状分布绕腰一圈故名。主要是由湿热内蕴,肝胆热甚,感受热毒之邪。初起患处有刺痛,局部皮肤潮红。水疱皮损有如黄豆或绿豆大,皮损分界清楚,水疱排列如带状。起初水疱壁厚,疱内液体透亮,五六日后变混浊,约10天后渐加干燥结痂而不留瘢痕。少数患者疼痛持续较长时间。

Herpes zoster mainly in the lumbar and hypochondriac regions with small red vesicles like beads forming a girdle around the waist. It is mostly caused by endogenous damp heat, hyperactivity of fire in the liver and gallbladder or affection of exogenous toxin. At the onset there is stabbing pain of the affected skin, which soon becomes erythematous. Patches of blisters in the size of mump-beans or soybeans are evolved, forming a bandlike distribution with clear cut interspaces btween the patches. The blisters are thick-walled and their contents are transparent at first, but turn turbid in five to six days. Resolution of the cutaneous lesions after decrustation without scar formation occurs in about ten days. In some cases pain lasts longer.

3.2.2 治疗
3.2.2 Treatment

首先要分带状疱疹的头和尾,首先出现皮损的部位是头部,然后延伸尾端的部位叫尾部。以三棱针点刺出血:点刺数次带状疱疹头部,点刺数次其尾部,及在其周围点刺数次。然后针:曲池、血海、委中、阳陵泉、太冲,施以泻法。

Firstly, the head and the tail of the location of herpes zoster should be distinguished, The area where the skin lesions first appeared is considered as the tail, while the extending part of herpes as the head of its locality. Prick the skin around herpes zoster with the a three edges needle to cause a little bleeding, several times at the head of the herpes zoster area and then several times at the tail, and also several pricks along both sides.

Then select and needle Quchi(LI 11), Xuehai(SP 10), Weizhong(BL 40) Yanglingquan(GB 34), and Taichong(LR 3) with reducing method.

3.3 耳聋、耳鸣
3.3 Deafness and Tinnitus

两者均属听力障碍。耳鸣为病人自觉耳中鸣响;耳聋则为听力减退或丧失听力。两者在病因及治疗上有其相似之处,故此合并讨论。

Both deafness and tinnitus are auditory disturbances. Tinnitus is characterized by ringing sound in the ears felt by the patient and deafness is failing or loss of hearing. Because of the similarities between these two conditions in etiology and treatment, they are discussed together.

3.3.1 辨证
3.3.1 Differentiation

3.3.1.1 实证
3.3.1.1 Excess type

主要表现：暴聋,或耳胀耳鸣,压之不减。肝胆风火上扰者有面红,口干,烦躁易怒,脉弦有力；风邪外袭者可有头痛,脉浮。

Main manifestations: Sudden deafness, or distension sensation and ringing in the ear that can not be eliminated by pressing. In the cases of upward rising of pathogenic wind fire of the liver and gallbladder, there are flushed face, dry mouth, irritability and hot temper, forceful and string taut pulse. In the case of invasion by exogenous pathogenic wind, headache and superficial pulse, may happen.

3.3.1.2 虚证
3.3.1.2 Deficiency type

主要表现：久病耳聋,或耳鸣时作时止,劳累加剧,按之则减,头晕,腰酸痛,遗精,白带多,脉细弱。

Main manifestation: Protracted deafness, intermittent tinnitus aggravated by strain and eliminated by pressing, dizziness, soreness and aching of the lower back, seminal emission, excessive leukorrhea, thready and weak pulse.

3.3.2 治疗
3.3.2 Treatmetn

主要选取手足少阳经穴位。实则泻之,虚则补之,也可加灸。
处方:翳风、听会、侠溪、中渚、足临泣。
实证:肝胆火盛加针外关、合谷;虚证:加肾俞、命门、太溪。

Points of Shaoyang meridians of Hand and Foot are used as the principal points. The reducing method is applied for excess condition, while the reinforcing for deficiency conditoon. Moxibustion is also advisable.

Prescription : Yifeng(SJ 17), Tinghui(GB 2), Xiaxi(GB 43), Zhongzhu(SJ 3).

Excessive fire in the liver and gallbladder channels: Xingjian(LR 2), Zulingqi(GB 41).

Invasion of exogenous pathogenic wind: Waiguan(SJ 5), Hegu(LI 4):

Deficiency of the kidney: Shenshu(BL 23), Mingmen (DU 4), Taixi(KI 3).

3.4 目赤肿痛
3.4 Congestion, Swelling and Pain of the Eye

3.4.1 辨证
3.4.1 Differentiation

主要表现:目赤肿痛,羞明流泪,眵多。风热者兼见发热,脉浮数;肝胆火盛可见口苦,烦热,便秘,脉弦。

Main manifestations: Congestion, swelling and pain of the eye, photophobia, lacrimation and sticky discharge. In the cases of wind heat, there aer fever, superficial and rapid pulse. In the case of excessive fire in the liver and gallbladder channels, there are bitter taste in the mouth, irritability with feverish sensation, constipation and string—taut pulse.

3.4.2 治疗
3.4.2 Treatment

近端取穴和远端配穴相结合以疏散风热之邪。施以泻法。
处方:睛明、风池、太阳、合谷、行间。
风热外邪加针外关;肝胆火盛加针太冲。

Distal and local points are used in combination to disperse wind heat. Needling is given with the reducing method.

Prescription: Jingming(BL 1), Fengchi(GB 20), Taiyang(EX-HN 15), Hegu(LI 4), Xingjian(LR 2)

Wind heat invasion: Waiguan(SJ 5).

Excessive fire in the liver and gallbladder channels: Taichong(LR 3).

该症包括现代医学之急性结膜炎、假膜性结膜炎及红眼病等病。

This condition is involved in acute conjunctivitis, pseudomenbranous conjunctivitis, epidemic kerato-conjunctivitis, etc, in modern medicine.

3.5 鼻渊
3.5 Thick and Sticky Nasal Discharge

3.5.1 辨证
3.5.1 Differentiation

主要表现:鼻塞,不闻香臭,黄臭浊涕;伴见咳嗽,前额隐隐作痛,舌红苔白腻,脉数。

Main manifestations: Nasal obstruction, loss of the sense of smell, yellow fetid nasal discharge, thick and sticky, accompanied by cough, dull pain in the forehead, rapid pulse, reddened tongue with thin, white and sticky coating.

3.5.2 治疗
3.5.2 Treatment

选取手太阴及手阳明经穴为主以宣肺气、疏散风热之邪。针以泻法。

处方:列缺、迎香、合谷、印堂。

Points of the hand Taiyin and hand Yangming meridians are selected as the principal ones to smooth the flow of the lung Qi and expel pathogenic wind heat by applying the reducing method.

prescription: Lieque(LU-7), Yingxiang(L1-20), Hegu(Li-4), Yintang(EX-HN 3).

本病相当于现代医学之慢性鼻炎、鼻窦炎。

The condition corresponds to chronic rhinitis and chronic nasosinusitis in modern medicine.

3.6 鼻衄
3.6 Epistaxis

3.6.1 辨证
3.6.1 Differentiation

3.6.1.1 **肺胃热盛**
3.6.1.1 **Extreme heat in lung and stomach**

主要表现：鼻衄，伴见发热，咳嗽，舌红，脉滑数；或见口渴喜冷饮，便秘，口臭，舌红苔黄，脉数有力。

Main manifestations: Epistaxis accompanied by fever, cough, reddened tongue, superficial and rapid pulse; or thirst with preference for cold drinking, constipation, foul breath, yellow coating, red tongue forceful and rapid pulse.

3.6.1.2 **阴虚火旺**
3.6.1.2 **Hyperactivity of fire due to deficiency of Yin**

主要表现：鼻衄，伴见面色潮红，口咽干燥，五心烦热，午后潮热，盗汗，脉细数。

Main manifestations: Epistaxis accompanied by malar flush, dryness of the mouth, feverish sensation of the palms and soles, afternoon fever, night sweating, thready and rapid pulse.

3.6.2 治疗
3.6.2 Treatment

处方：迎香、合谷、上星。

肺热者加少商；胃热者加内庭；阴虚火旺加照海穴。实则泻之，虚则补之。

Prescription：Yingxiang(LI 20), Hegu(LI 4), Shangxing(DU 23).
Supplementary points：
Heat in the lung：Shaoshang(LU 11).
Heat in the stomach：Neiting(ST 44).
Hyperaltivity of fire due to deficiency of Yin ：Zhaohai(KI 6).
Reducing method for excessive heat and reinforcing for cleficient heat.

鼻衄可因肿瘤、鼻部疾病或急性发热性疾病引起。除了针刺治疗之外，须依原发病不同而采用其他治疗方法。

Epistaxis may be caused by trauma, nasal disorders and acute febrile diseases. In addition to acupuncture treatment, other therapeutic measures should be adopted according to its primary cause.

3.7 牙痛
3.7 Toothache

3.7.1 辨证
3.7.1 Differentiantion

3.7.1.1 胃火

3.7.1.1 Stoamch fire

主要表现:剧烈牙痛,口臭,口干,便秘,舌苔黄,脉数有力。

Main manifestations: Severe toothache accompanied by foul breath, thirst, constipation, yellow tongue coating, forceful and rapid pulse.

3.7.1.2 风火
3.7.1.2 Wind fire

主要表现:急性牙痛,牙龈肿胀,伴见发热恶寒,脉浮数。

Main manifestations: Acute toothache with gingival swelling accompanied by chills and fever, superficial and rapid pulse.

3.7.1.3 肾阴虚
3.7.1.3 Deficiency of the Kidney Yin

主要表现:牙痛隐隐,时作时止,牙齿浮动,口无臭味,舌质红,脉细数。

Main manifestations: Dull pain off and on, loose teeth, absence of foul breath, reddened tongue, thready and rapid pulse.

3.7.2 治疗
3.7.2 Treatment

3.7.2.1 胃火
3.7.2.1 Stomach fire

处方:合谷、颊车、内庭、下关。

针以泻法。

Prescription: Hegu(LI 4), Jiache(ST 6), Neiting(ST 44), Xiaguan(ST 37).

Apply reducing method.

3.7.2.2 风火

3.7.2.2 Wind fire
处方：耳门、风池、合谷、颊车、下关、外关。
针以泻法。

Prescription: Yemen(SJ 2), Fengchi(GB 20), Hegu(LI 4), Jiache(ST 6), Xianguan(ST 7), Waiguan(SJ 5), Needle them with reducing method.

3.7.2.3 肾阴虚
3.7.2.3 Deficiency of Kidney Yin
处方：颊车、下关、太溪。
针以补法。

Prescription: Jiache(ST 6), Xiaguan(ST 7), Taixi(KI 3). Needle them with reinforcing method.

3.8 咽喉痛
3.8 Sore Throat

3.8.1 辨证
3.8.1 Differentiation

3.8.1.1 实热证
3.8.1.1 Syndrome of excess of heat

主要表现：起病突然,恶寒,发热,头痛,咽喉肿痛,口渴,吞咽不利,便秘,舌质红苔黄,脉浮数,此为风热在表。热邪在里者但热不寒,脉滑数。

Main manifestations: Abrupt onset with chills, fever, headache, congested and sore throat, thirst, dysphagia, constipation, reddened

199

tongue with thin yellow coating, superficial and rapid pulse. These are the symptoms of exterior wind heat syndrome. In case of excess interior heat syndrome, patient may have fever without chills, and rolling and rapid pulse.

3.8.1.2 阴虚证
3.8.1.2 Syndrome of deficiency of Yin

主要表现:渐渐起病,无热或低热,咽喉稍红肿,时有疼痛,或吞咽时痛,咽干,夜间尤甚,五心烦热,舌红无苔,脉细数。

Main manifestations: Gradual onset without fever or with low fever, slightly congested throat with intermittent pain or pain during swallowing, dryness of the throat, more marked at night, feverish sensation in the palms and soles, reddened and furless tongue, thready and rapid pulse.

3.8.2 治疗
3.8.2 Treatment

3.8.2.1 实热证
3.8.2.1 Excess of heat

处方:少商、合谷、内庭、天容。

针施以泻法。

Prescription: Shaoshang(LU 11), Hegu(LI 4), Neiting(ST 44), Tianrong(SI 17). Needle them with reducing method.

3.8.2.2 阴虚证
3.8.2.2 Deficiency of Yin

处方:①太溪、鱼际、廉泉;②照海、列缺、扶突。

两方可交替使用。

针施以补泻并用。

Prescription: (a) Taixi(KI 3), Yuji(LU 10), Lianquan(RN 23) (b) Zhaohai(KI 6), Lieque(LU 7), Futu(LI 18). Needle them with reinforcing method.

The above two prescriptions (a) and (b) may be used alternatively.

3.9 视神经萎缩
3.9 Optic Atrophy

3.9.1 辨证
3.9.1 Differentiation

3.9.1.1 肝肾阴虚
3.9.1.1 Deficiency of liver and kidney Yin

主要表现:眼睛干涩,视物模糊,头晕耳鸣,梦遗腰酸,舌红少苔,脉细弱。

Main manifestationsa: Dryness of the the eyes, blurred vision, dizziness, tinnitus, nocturnal emission, aching of the lower back reddened tongue with scanty coating, thready and weak pule.

3.9.1.2 气血不足
3.9.1.2 Deficiency of Qi and blood

主要表现:眼花,气短懒言,倦怠纳呆,便溏,舌淡苔薄白,脉细弱。

Main manifestaitons: Blurred vision, weakness of breath, disinclination to talk, lassitude, poor appetite, loose stools, pale tongue with thin white coating thready and weak pulse.

3.9.1.3 肝气郁结
3.9.1.3 Stagnation of liver Qi

主要表现：视物昏花，精神抑郁，头目眩晕，胁痛，口苦咽干，脉弦。

Main manifestations: Blurred vision, emotional depression, dizziness, vertigo, hypochondriac pain, bitter taste in the mouth, dry throat and string—taut pulse.

3.9.2 治疗
3.9.2 Treatment

对肝肾阴虚、气血不足者主要选取少阴、太阳经穴，施以补法以滋养肝肾，补益气血。对于肝气郁结者可施以平补平泻法以疏肝解郁。

处方：风池、睛明、光明。

肝肾阴虚加太冲、太溪、肝俞、肾俞；

气血不足加足三里、三阴交；

肝气郁结者加针期门、太冲、阳陵泉。

To reinforce the liver and kidney and nourish Qi and blood by puncturing the points in the Foot—Shaoyang and Taiyang meridian with reinforcing method for deficiency of the liver and kidney Yin, and deficiency of Qi and blood. Even method is used to same points to remove the sagnation of liver Qi.

Prescription: Fengchi(GB 20), Jingming(BL 1), Guangming(GB 39).

Deficiency of liver and kidney Yin: Taichong(LR 3), Taixi(KI 3), Ganshu(BL 18), Shenshu(BL 23).

Deficiency of Qi and blood: Zusanli(ST 36), Sanyinjiao(Sp 6).

Stagnation of liver Qi: Qimen (LR 14), Taichong (LR 3), Yanglingquan (GB 34).

第四章 其他病症
CHAPTER FOUR
MISCELLANEOUS DISEASES

4.1 粉刺
4.1 Acne

4.1.1 辨证
4.1.1 Differentiation

4.1.1.1 肺经风热
4.1.1.1 Type of Wind Heat in Lungs

主要表现:颜面潮红,粉刺燉热,疼痛,或有脓疱,舌红苔薄黄,脉数而浮。

Main manifestations : Flushed complexion, pain and hot sensation in acne, pustule, red tongue and thin yellow coating, superficial and rapid pulse.

4.1.1.2 肠胃湿热
4.1.1.2 Type of Dampness Heat in Stomach and Intestines

主要表现:皮疹红肿疼痛,伴有便秘,尿黄,纳呆,腹胀,舌红苔黄腻,脉滑数。

Main manifestations: Redish and painful acne , constipation, yellowish urine, anorexia, abdominal distension, yellow sticky tongue coating, slippery and rapid pulse.

4.1.1.3 脾失健运
4.1.1.3 Type of Dysfunction of Spleen

主要表现：皮疹色红不鲜，反复发作，或伴纳呆、便溏、神疲，舌苔薄白，脉濡数。

Main manifestations: Redish acne and recuring, accompanied by poor appetite, loose stool, lassitude, thin white coating, soft and superficial, rapid pulse.

4.1.1.4 瘀血阻滞
4.1.1.4 Type of Blood Stagnation

主要表现：粉刺日久不愈，皮疹暗黑，有结节，舌暗苔薄白，脉弦。

Main manifestations: Protracted acne and dark in color, dark and red tongue with thin white coating, string—taut pulse.

4.1.1.5 肝肾不足
4.1.1.5 Type of Liver and Kidney Deficiency

主要表现：粉刺鲜红，伴有腰膝酸软，舌淡红，苔薄白，或少苔，脉细。

Main manifestations: Fresh red acne in the femal, accompanied by sore low back and knees, pink tongue and thin white coating or scanty coating, thready pulse.

4.1.2 治疗
4.1.2 Treatment

4.1.2.1 肺经风热
4.1.2.1 Type of Wind Heat in Lungs

治法：疏风清热宣肺。

处方：尺泽、合谷、大椎、肺俞。

操作：尺泽、合谷、大椎均用毫针泻法。肺俞先用三棱针点刺，然后再拔火罐。

Principle of treatment: Disperssing the lungs and clearing off heat

Points: Chize (LU 5), Dazhui (DU 14), Hegu (L1 4), Feishu (BL 13).

Manipulation: Apply reducing in LU 5, DU 14 and LI 4 with filiform needle. Apply pricking puncture in BL13 then cupping.

4.1.2.2 肠胃湿热
4.1.2.2 Type of Dampness Heat in Stomach and Intestines

治法：清热化湿通腑。

处方：曲池、上巨墟、天枢、阴陵泉。

操作：毫针泻法。

Principle of treatment: Clearing off heat, promoting diuresis and purgating the intestines.

Points: Quchi (LI 11), Shangjuxu (ST 37), Tianshu (ST 25), Yinlingquan (SP 9)

Manipulation: Apply reducing method with filiform needle.

4.1.2.3 脾失健运
4.1.2.3 Type of Dysfunction of Spleen

治法：健脾化湿。

处方：三阴交、足三里、合谷、脾俞。

操作：毫针补法，可灸。

Principle of Treatment: Replenishing spleen to promote diuresis

Points: Sanyinjiao (SP 6), Zusanli (ST 36), Hegu (LI 4), Pishu (BL 20).

Manipulation: Apply reinforcing method, or moxibustion.

4.1.2.4 瘀血阻滞

4.1.2.4 **Type of Blood Stagnation**

治法:活血化瘀,养颜。

处方:膈俞、内关、四关穴、血海、肺俞。

操作:除肺俞、膈俞刺络拔罐外,其余各穴均用毫针泻法。

Principle of treatment: Activating the blood circulation and removing blood stasis

Points: Geshu(BL 17), Neiguan(PC 6), Four—gate points(LI4 and LR3), Xuehai(SP 10), Feishu(BL 13)

Manipulation: Apply pricking puncture with three-edged needle and cupping in BL 13 and BL 17; apply reducing method in other points with filiform needles.

4.1.2.5 肝肾不足

4.1.2.5 **Type Deficiency of Live and Kidney**

治法:补益肝肾。

处方:太溪、三阴交、曲泉、肝俞、肾俞。

操作:毫针补法。

Principle of treatment: Invigorating Kidney and Liver.

Points: Taixi(KI 3), Sanyinjiao(SP 6), Ququan(LR 8), Ganshu(BL 18), Shenshu(BL 23).

Manipulation: Apply reinforcing method with filiform needles.

4.2 肥胖症
4.2 Obesity

4.2.1 辨证

4.2.1 Differentiation

4.2.1.1 脾胃旺盛

4.2.1.1 Hyperactivity of Spleen and Stomach

主要表现:形体肥胖,上下匀称,肌肉坚实,食欲亢进,面色红润,畏热多汗,腹胀,便秘,舌质正常或偏红,舌苔薄黄,脉滑有力。

Main manifestations: Obesity, even shape, well—built, polyorexia, redish and lustrous complexion, intolerance to hot, much sweating, abdominal fullness, constipation, normal or red tongue, thin yellow coating, slippery and forceful pulse.

4.2.1.2 脾胃俱虚

4.2.1.2 Deficiency of Spleen and Stomach

主要表现:体胖,以面、颈部为甚,肌肉松弛,面色苍白,神疲乏力,形寒怕冷,纳呆腹胀,便秘,或尿少浮肿,舌淡苔薄白,脉沉细而迟。

Main manifestations: Obesity, especially on the face and of nap region, feeble muscle, pale complexion, lassitude, intolerance to cold, cold limbs, poor appetite, abdominal fullness and constipation, or edema, and decreased output of urine, pale tongue, thin and white coating, deep and thready pulse.

4.2.1.3 真元不足

4.2.1.3 Deficiency of Essence

主要表现:肥胖,以臀、大腿部为甚,肌肉松弛,神疲乏力,喜静恶动,面色㿠白,纳可或偏少,易畏寒,或尿少浮肿,舌淡有齿痕,苔薄白,脉沉细。

Main manifestations: Obesity, especially of hips and thigh, feeble muscle, lassitude, dislike to exercise and desire for rest, pale comeplexion, normal appetite or slightly poor appetite, intolerance to cold, or decreased urine and edema, pale tongue with teeth marks, thin and white coating, deep and thready pulse.

4.2.2 治疗

4.2.2 Treatment

4.2.2.1 脾胃旺盛

4.2.2.1 Hyperactivity of Spleen and Stomach

治法：泻脾胃、抑亢进。

处方：商丘、梁丘、内庭、天枢。

操作：毫针泻法。

Principle of treatment：Reducing the spleen and stomach to inhibit the appetite.

Points：Shanqiu(SP 5), Liangqiu(ST 34), Neiting(ST 44) Tianshu (ST 25).

Manipulation：Apply reducing method with filiform needle.

4.2.2.2 脾胃俱虚

4.2.2.2 Deficienency of Spleen and Stomach

治法：健脾运胃、减肥。

处方：太白、足三里、丰隆、脾俞、天枢。

操作：太白、足三里、脾俞可用补法；天枢、丰隆平补平泻；脾俞亦可灸。

Principle of treatment：Replenishing spleen and stomach to control weight.

Points：Taibai(SP 3), Zusanli(ST 36), Fenglong(ST 40), Pishu (BL 20), Tianshu(ST 25).

Manipulation：Apply reducind method in SP 3, ST 36 and BL 20; even method in ST 40 and ST 25; moxibustion in BL 20.

4.2.2.3 真元不足

4.2.2.3 Deficienency of Essence

治法：补益真元。

处方:太溪、关元、中脘、肾俞、三阴交、命门。
操作:毫针补法;可直接灸。

Principle of treatment: Replenishing the essence

Points: Taixi(KI 3), Guanyuan(RN 4) Zhongwan(RN 12), Shenshu(BL 23), Sanyinjiao(SP 6) Mingmen(DN 4)

Manipulation: Reinforcing method with filiform needle, or moxibustion.

4.3 雀斑
4.3 Freckle

4.3.1 辨证
4.3.1 Differentiation

4.3.1.1 肝肾不足
4.3.1.1 Deficiency of Kidney and Liver

主要表现:面部雀斑,色淡黄,月经期色变深,腰膝酸软,舌淡红苔薄白,脉细。

Main manifestations: Facial freckle, sallow in color, becoming dark during the menstrual period, sore and weak of knees and low back, pale tongue, thin and white coating, thready pulse.

4.3.1.2 气滞血瘀
4.3.1.2 Stagnation of Blood and Qi

主要表现:面部雀斑,色淡黑,情绪波动时变深,舌暗脉弦。

Main manifestations: Blackish freckle, becoming darker in unusual reaction of emotions, dark tongue, string—taut pulse.

4.3.2 治疗
4.3.2 Treatment

4.3.2.1 肝肾不足
4.3.2.1 Deficiency of Kidney and Liver

治法:补益肝肾祛斑。

处方:肝俞、肾俞、大椎、内关、颧髎。

操作:毫针补法。

Principle of treatment: Invigorating the Kidney and Liver to remove the freckle.

Points: Ganshu(BL 18), Shenshu(BL 23), Dazhui(DU 14), Neiguan(PC 6), Quanliao(ST 18).

Manipulation: Apply reinforcing method with filiform needle.

4.3.2.2 气滞血瘀
4.3.2.2 Stagnation of Blood and Qi

治法:行气活血祛瘀。

处方:四关穴、血海、听宫、膈俞。

操作:毫针泻法。

Principle of treatment: Four — gate points (LI4 and LR3 bilateraly), Xuehai(SP 10), Tinggong(SI 19), Geshu(BL 17).

Manipulation: Apply reducing method with filiform needle.

4.4 美尼尔氏综合征
4.4 Meniere's Syndrome

4.4.1 辨证
4.4.1 Differentiation

4.4.1.1 肾虚髓亏
4.4.1.1 Insuficiency of Kidney and Marrow

主要表现:突发眩晕,耳鸣耳聋,发作频繁,神情萎靡,腰膝酸软,心烦失眠,手足心热,舌红少苔,脉弦细数。

Main manifestations: Sudden onset vertigo, tinnitus or deafness, frequently attack, accompanied by lassitude, sore and weak of knees and low back, restlessness and insomnia, feverish sensation in soles, palms and chest, red tongue and scanty coating, string—taut, thready and rapid pulse.

4.4.1.2 肝阳上亢
4.4.1.2 Hyperactivity of Liver yang

主要表现:眩晕因情绪波动而发,面赤头痛,口苦咽干,目赤,胸胁胀满,舌红苔黄,脉弦数。

Main manifestations: Vertigo, often induced by unusual emotional reactions, flushed face, headache, bitter taste in the mouth, dry throat, redish eyes, fullness in hypochondriac region, red tongue, yellow coating, string—taut pulse.

4.4.1.3 寒水上泛

4.4.1.3 Upwards Attack of Pathogenic Cold Fluid

主要表现：眩晕,心下悸动,咳嗽痰稀,腰痛背冷,尿清长,舌淡苔白润,脉沉细弱。

Main manifestations: Vertigo, throbbing feeling in epigastric region, cough with clear sputum, pain and cold sensation in low back, cold limbs, clear urine and increasing output, pale tongue, white and moist coating, deep thready and weak pulse.

4.4.1.4 痰浊中阻
4.4.1.4 Accumulation of Phlegm and Turbid Fluid in Middle Warmer

主要表现：眩晕,头重痛,胸闷,呕恶痰多,纳呆倦怠,舌苔白腻,脉濡或滑。

Main manifestations: Vertigo, headache with a heavy sensation, fullness in chest, vomiting or nausea with sputum, lost of appetite, lassitude, whtie and sticky tongue coating, superficial soft or slippery pulse.

4.4.2 治疗
4.4.2 Treatment

4.4.2.1 肾髓亏虚
4.4.2.1 Insufficiency of Kidney and Liver

治法：滋肾生髓定眩。

处方：听会、太溪。

操作：补太溪,平补平泻听会。

Principle of treatment: Invigorating the kidney, replenishing the marrow to relieve virtigo.

Points: Tinghui(GB 2), Taixi(KI 3).

Manipulation: Apply even method in GB 2; reinforcing in KI 3.

4.4.2.2 肝阳上亢

4.4.2.2 **Hyperactivity of Liver Yang**

治法:平肝潜阳熄风。

处方:四关穴、听会。

操作:毫针泻法。

Principle of treatment:Calming the liver to inhibit the endogenous wind.

Points:Four—gate points(LI 4 and LR 3 bilateraly),Tinghui(GB 2).

Manipulation:Apply reducing method with filiform needle.

4.4.2.3 寒水上泛

4.4.2.3 **Upwards Attack of pathogenic Cold Fluid**

治法:温化寒水。

处方:中脘、水分、听会。

操作:针听会穴,中脘、水分以艾灸。

Principle of treatment:Warming the Yang and resolving the pathogenic cold fluid.

Points:Zhongwan(RN 12),Shuifen(RN 9),Tinghui(GB 2).

Manlpulation:Apply needling in GB 2,moxibustion in RN 9 and RN 12.

4.4.2.4 痰浊中阻

4.4.2.4 **Accumulation of Phlegm and Turbid Fluid in Middle Warmer**

治法:祛痰浊定眩晕。

处方:百会、丰隆、听会、中脘。

操作:用灸法。

Principle of treatment:Resolving the phlegm and turbid fluid to relieve vertigo.

Polnts:Baihui(Du 20),Fenglong(ST 40),Tinghui(GB 2),Zhongwan(RN 12).

Manipulation: Moxibustion.

4.5 高脂血症
4.5 Hyperlipemia

4.5.1 辨证
4.5.1 Differentiation

4.5.1.1 脾肾阳虚
4.5.1.1 Yang Deficiency in Both Spleen and Kidney

主要表现:面色㿠白,乏力神倦,畏寒肢冷,纳减便溏,甚或五更泄泻,尿少肢肿,舌淡胖有齿印,脉沉细弱。

Main manifestations: Pale complexion, lassitude, cold limbs and intolerance to cold, poor appetite and loose stools, or diarrhoea at dawn in severe cases, decreased urine and edema in lower extremities, pale and swollen tongue with teeth marks, deep thready and weak pulse.

4.5.1.2 肝肾阴虚
4.5.1.2 Yin Insufficiency of kidney and Liver

主要表现:头晕,耳鸣,腰膝酸软,咽干少寐,颧红盗汗,五心烦热,遗精,舌红少苔,脉细数。

Main manifestations: Dizziness and tinnitus, sore and weak knees and low back, dry throat, insomnia, flushed cheek, nocturnal sweating, nocturnal emission, feverish sensation in palms, soles and in chest, red tongue and scanty coating, thready and rapid pulse.

4.5.1.3 痰浊内阻

4.5.1.3 Obstruction of phlegm and Turbid Fluid

主要表现:头晕,胸闷脘痞,纳呆便溏,肢体沉重,苔白腻,脉弦或滑。

Main manifestations: Fullness in chest and epigastric region, dizziness and distending sensation of head, heavy sensation of body, white and sticky coating, string—taut or slippery pulse.

4.5.1.4 气滞血瘀
4.5.1.4 Stagnation of Blood and Qi

主要表现:胁肋胀痛,心悸胸闷,胸痛彻背,舌暗,脉涩。

Main manifestations: Fullness in hypochondriac region, palpitation, pain in the chest radiating to the back, dark tongue, hesitant pulse.

4.5.2 治疗
4.5.2 Treatment

4.5.2.1 脾肾阳虚
4.5.2.1 Yang Deflciency in Both Spleen and kidney

治法:温补脾肾。

处方:脾俞、肾俞、中脘、关元、丰隆。

操作:艾灸。

Principle of treatment: Invigorating the spleen and Kidney.

Points: Pishu(BI 20), Shenshu(BL 20), Zhongwan(RN 12), Guanyuan(RN 3), Fenglong(ST 40).

Manipulation: Moxibustion.

4.5.2.2 肝肾阴虚
4.5.2.2 Yin Insufficiency of Kidney and Liver

治法:滋养肝肾。

处方:肝俞、肾俞、太溪、三阴交、蠡沟。
操作:施以毫针补法。

Principle of treatment: Nourishing the liver and kidney.

Points: Ganshu(BL 18), Shenshu(BL 23), Taixi(KI 3), Sanyinjiao(SP 6), Ligou(LR 5).

Manipulation: Apply reinforcing method of acupuncture.

4.5.2.3 痰浊内阻
4.5.2.3 Obstruction of Phlegm and Turbid Fluid

治法:健脾化痰浊。
处方:公孙、内关、丰隆、中脘。
操作:针以泻法。

Princile of treatment: Invigorating spleen to resolove the phlegm and turbid fluid.

Points: Gongsun(SP 4), Neiguan(PC 6), Fenglong(ST 40), Zhongwan(RN 12).

Manipulation: Apply reducing method of acupuncture.

4.5.2.4 气滞血瘀
4.5.2.4 Stagnation of Blood and Qi

治法:行气活血化瘀。
处方:四关穴、血海、心俞、膈俞、内关。
操作:施以毫针泻法。

Principle of treatment: Activating blood circulation and removing the blood stasis.

Points: Four—gate points(LI 4 and LR 3 bilateraly), Xuehai(SP 10), xinshu(BL 15), Geshu(BL 17), Neiguan(PC 6).

Manipulation: Apply reducing method of acupuncture.

4.6 结肠激惹综合征
4.6 Irritable Colon Syndrome

4.6.1 辨证
4.6.1 Differentiation

4.6.1.1 湿热下注
4.6.1.1 Downwards Attack of Dampness Heat Evil
主要表现:发热,腹痛腹泻,里急后重,大便不爽,苔腻,脉滑。

Main manifestations: Fever, abdominal pain, diarrhoea, rectal tenesemus, unsmooth defecation, sticky tongue coating, slippery pulse.

4.6.1.2 肝旺脾虚
4.6.1.2 Liver Qi Stagnation and Deficiency of Spleen Qi
主要表现:怒后腹痛肠鸣,泻后痛减,脘闷纳少,胸胁胀痛,苔薄白,脉弦细。

Main manifestations: Abdominal pain and borborygmi, especially after a fit of angery, pain relieved after bowel movement, fullness in epigastric region, poor appetite, distending pain in hypochondriac region, white and thin coating of tongue, thready and string-taut pulse.

4.6.1.3 脾胃虚弱
4.6.1.3 Deficiency of Spleen and Stomach
主要表现:腹泻肠鸣,缠绵不愈,完谷不化,纳呆脘闷,乏力,舌淡苔白,脉濡缓。

Main manifestations: Diarrhoea, borborygmi, prolonged and intractable, undigested food in stools, poor appetite, full sensation in the chest, lassitude, pale tongue and white coating, superficial, soft and even slow pulse.

4.6.1.4 肾阳虚衰
4.6.1.4 Deficiency of Kidney Yang

主要表现：五更泄泻,肠鸣腹痛,迁延日久不愈,畏寒面白,腰膝酸软,苔白,脉沉细而无力。

Main manifestations: Diarrhoea at dawn, borborygmi, abdominal pain, difficult to be cured, intolerance to cold, pale complexion, sore and weak knees and low back, white tongue coating, deep, thready and weak pulse.

4.6.2 治疗
4.6.2 Treatment

4.6.2.1 湿热下注
4.6.2.1 Downwards Attack of Dampness Heat Evil
治法：清利湿热。
处方：曲池、阴陵泉、天枢、大肠俞、外关、上巨墟。
操作：施以泻法。

Principle of treatment: Promoting diuresis and clearing off heat.
Points: Quchi (LI 11), Yinlingquan (SP 9), Tianshu (ST 25), Dachangshu (BL 25), Waiguan (SJ 5), Shangjuxu (ST 37).
Manipulation: Apply reducing method with filiform needle.

4.6.2.2 肝旺脾虚
4.6.2.2 Liver Qi Stagnation and Deficiency of Spleen Qi
治法：抑肝实脾。
处方：太冲、大都、脾俞、足三里、肝俞、期门。
操作：太冲、肝俞、期门施以泻法,大都、足三里、脾俞施以补法。

Principle of treatment: Disperssing stagnated liver energy and invigorating spleen Qi.

Points: Taichong (LR 3), Dadu (SP 2), Pishu (BL 20), Zusanli (ST 36), Ganshu (BL 18), Qimen (LR 14)

Manipulation: Apply reducing method in LR 3, BL 18, and LR 14; reinforcing method in BL 20, ST 36 and SP 2

4.6.2.3. 脾胃虚弱
4.6.2.3 Deficiency of Spleen and Stomach.
治法：健运脾胃。
处方：脾俞、胃俞、中脘、足三里、天枢。
操作：针以补法，可灸。

Principle of treatment: Invigorating the spleen and stomach.

Points: Pishu (BL 20), Weishu (BL 21), Zhongwan (RN 12), Zusanli (ST 36), Tianshu (ST 25).

Manipulation: Apply reinforcing method of acupuncture or moxibustion.

4.6.2.4. 肾阳虚衰
4.6.2.4. Deficiency of Kidney Yang
治法：温肾止泻。
处方：神阙、关元、肾俞、足三里、命门。
操作：针以补法加灸。

Principle of treatment: Invigorating kidney Yang to stop diarrhoea.

Points: Shenque (RN 8), Guanyuan (RN 3), Shenshu (BL 32), Zusanli (ST 36), Mingmen (DU 4).

Manipulation: Apply reinforcing method of acupuncture or moxibustion.

4.7 前列腺炎
4.7 Prostatitis

4.7.1 辨证
4.7.1 Differentiation

4.7.1.1 湿热下注
4.7.1.1 Downwards Attack of Dampness Heat Evil

主要表现：小便混浊或夹凝块，尿道灼热感，尿中带血，口渴，会阴部胀痛，舌红苔黄腻，脉滑数。

Mani manifestations: Cloudy urine or with clot, urethral burning, blood in urine, thirsty, fullness and pain in perineurium, red tongue and yellow sticky coating, slippery and rapid pulse.

4.7.1.2 脾虚气陷
4.7.1.2 Deficiency of Spleen Qi and Prolapse of Qi in Middle Warme

主要表现：小便混浊，反复发作，经久不愈，小腹坠胀，面色无华，神疲，舌淡苔白，脉沉细。

Main manifestation: Cloudy urine, recuring, diffcult to be cured, empty feeling and fullness in lower abdomen, pale complexion, lassitude, pale tongue and white coating, deep and thready pulse.

4.7.1.3 下元虚衰
4.7.1.3 Depletion of Lower Yuan (Source)

主要表现：小便淋漓，兼有白浊，迁延日久，腰膝疲软，畏寒肢冷，舌淡苔白，脉沉。

Main manifestations: Dribbling in urination, or white cloudy urine, prolonged and difficult to be cured, sore and weak knees and low back, intolerance to cold and cold limbs, pale tongue and white coating, deep pulse.

4.7.1.4 气滞血瘀
4.7.1.4 Stagnation of Blood and Qi

主要表现:会阴酸胀疼痛,分泌物少,腺体硬化,舌暗有瘀斑,脉弦涩。

Main manifestations: Fullness and pain in perineurium, scanty secretion and sclerosis which are found in prostate gland check, dark purplish tongue with petechia, string-taut pulse.

4.7.2 治疗
4.7.2 Treatment

4.7.2.1 湿热下注
4.7.2.1 Downwards Attack of Dampness Heat Evil

治法:清利湿热。
处方:中极、阴陵泉、膀胱俞、三阴交。
操作:针以泻法。

Principle of treatment: Clearing off heat and promoting diuresis.

Points: Zhongji(RN 3), Yinlingquan(SP 9), Pangguanshu (BL 28), Sanyinjiao(SP 6).

Manipulation: Apply reducing method with filiform needle.

4.7.2.2 脾虚气陷
4.7.2.2 Deficiency of Spleen Qi and Prolapse of Qi in Middle Warme

治法:健脾益气。
处方:三阴交、气海、足三里、脾俞、肾俞。
操作:针以补法加灸。

Principle of treatment: Invigorating spleen Qi.

Points: Sanyinjiao(SP 6), Qihai(RN 6), Zusanli(ST 36), Pishu (BL 20), Shenshu(BL 23).

Manipulation: Apply reinforcing method with filiform needle or moxibustion.

4.7.2.3 下元虚衰
4.7.2.3 Depletion of Lower Yuan (Source)

治法：温补下元。

处方：关元、三阴交、命门、肾俞。

操作：施以灸法。

Principle of treatment: Invigorating the lower Yuan(source) with warming treatment

Points: Guanyuan(RN 4), Sanyinjiao(SP 6), Mingmen(DU 4), Shenshu(BL 23)

Manipulation: Moxibustion

4.7.2.4 气滞血瘀
4.7.2.4 Stagnation of Blood and Qi

治法：行气活血化瘀。

处方：关元、太冲、次髎、归来、血海。

操作：针以泻法。

Principle of treatment: Activating the circulation of blood and removing blood stasis.

Points: Guanyuan(RN 4), Taichong(LR 3), Ciliao(BL 32), Guilai(ST 29), Xuehai(SP 10).

Manipulation: Apply reducing method with filiform needle.

第五章 急症处理
CHAPTER FIVE
THE TREATMENT OF EMERGENCIES

5.1 厥脱
5.1 Syncope

5.1.1 辨证
5.1.1 Differentiation

5.1.1.1 实证
5.1.1.1 Excessive Syndrome

主要表现：突然昏仆不省人事，牙关紧闭，两手握拳，身热烦躁，面红气粗，喉中痰鸣或手足厥冷，脉沉弦或沉滑有力。

Main manifestations: Sudden fainting and loss of consciousness, clenched jaws and tightly closed hands, fever and restlessness, flushed face, coarse breathing, rattling in the throat, or cold extremities, deep string-taut pulse.

5.1.1.2 虚证
5.1.1.2 Deficient Syndrome

主要表现：面色苍白，四肢厥冷，出冷汗，目陷睛迷，口张，手撒，甚则二便失禁，脉沉细或脉微欲绝。

Main manifestations: Pale complexion, extreme cold limbs, profuse cold sweating, blurred vision, agape mouth, flaccid open hands, incontinence of urine and feces in severe cases, deep thready or extreme weak pulse.

5.1.2 治疗
5.1.2 Treatment

5.1.2.1 实证
5.1.2.1 Excessive Syndrome

处方：人中、内关（双）、十二井穴。

针用泻法，十二井点刺放血。

口噤握拳，气粗肢冷者加针太冲；面红气粗，唇紫舌红，口噤握拳，脉沉者加针行间、涌泉；身热烦渴，脉沉伏而数者加大椎、曲池、合谷；喉中痰鸣声如拽锯，脉沉滑者加天突、丰隆、巨阙；兼有抽搐者加合谷、太冲、侠溪。

Prescription: Renzhong(DU 26), Neiguan(PC 6), Twelve Jing-(Well) points.

Puncture the points with the reducing method and let bleeding in twelve Jing-(well) points.

Supplementary points:

Clenched jaws, coarse breathing: Taichong(LR 3);

Flushed complexion, purplish lips, red tongue, clenched jaws and closed hands, and deep pulse: Dazhui(DU 14), Quchi(LI 11) and Hegu (LI 4);

Rattling in the throat and deep slippery pulse: Tiantu (RN 22), Fenglong(ST 40) and Juque (RN 14); and

Convulsions: Hegu(LI 4) and Xiaxi(GB 43).

5.1.2.2 虚证

5.1.2.2 Deficienct Syndrome

处方:百会、气海、关元、足三里。

上穴针后加灸或单用艾炷重灸。

面青身冷,卷卧肢冷,口不渴者加灸神阙;冷汗不止者加针复溜、合谷,并灸膻中;有大出血者可灸大敦;昏迷不醒者加针人中、合谷、内关。

Prescription: Baihui (DU 20), Qihai (RN 6), Guanyuan (RN 4) and Zusanli (ST 36).

Apply acupuncture and moxibustion or only intense moxibustion with moxa cons.

Supplementary points:

Greenish face and cold body, cold limbs and lassitude, no thirsty in mouth: Shenque (RN 8)

Profuse cold sweating: Puncture the Fuliu (KI 7), Hegu (LI 4) and apply moxibustion in Tangzhong (RN 17);

Syncope caused by severe loss of blood: Apply moxibustion in Dadun (LR 1); and

Loss of consciousness: Puncture Renzhong (DU 26), Hegu (LI 4) and Neiguan (PC 6).

5.2 惊厥抽搐
5.2 Convulsions

5.2.1 辨证
5.2.1 Differentiation

主要表现:全身或部分肌肉突然不自主地抽动或痉挛,伴有高热、项强,甚则角弓反张,昏迷、意识丧失。

Main manifestations: Convulsions or accompanied with high fever, stiffness of neck, or opisthotonus; coma, loss of consciousness in severe cases.

5.2.2 治疗
5.2.2 Treatment

处方:百会、风府、大椎、合谷、太冲、涌泉、十二井穴、人中、内关。

人中、十二井穴用三棱针刺血,其余诸穴针用泻法。

昏迷不醒加针人中;口噤不开加刺颊车、下关;上肢拘挛加针曲池、内关;下肢拘挛加针阳陵泉、承山;角弓反张加针风池、身柱;痰多加刺列缺、丰隆、膻中。

耳针:取神门、皮质下、枕、内分泌、肝穴。

针用泻法,留针30~60分钟。

Prescription: Baihui(DU 20), Fengfu(DU 16), Dazhui(DU 14), Hegu(KI 4), Taichong(LR 3), Yongquan(LI 1), Twelve Jing-(well) points, Neiguan(PC 6) and Renzhong(DU26).

Apply pricking puncture and let bleeding in DU 26 and 12 Jing-(well) points. Puncture the other points with reducing method.

Supplementary points:

Loss of consciousness: Renzhong(DU 26);

Clenched jaws: Jiache(ST 6) and Xiaguan(ST 7);

Muscular spasm in upper extremies: Quchi(LI 11) and Neiguan(PC 6);

Muscular spasm in lower extremies: Yanglingquan(GB 34) and Chenshang(BL 57);

Opithotonus: Fengchi(GB 20) and Shenzhu(DU 12);

Profuse sputum: Lieque(LU 9), Fenglong(ST 40) and Tangzhong(RN 17).

Auricular points: Shenmen, Subcortex, Occiput, Endocrine and Liver points.

Puncture the auricular points with filform needles and retain the needles for 30—60 minutes.

5.3 高热昏迷
5.3 Coma Due to High Fever

5.3.1 辨证
5.3.1 Differentiation

主要表现：腋下温度超过39℃，甚则超过41℃，严重者并见谵妄，昏迷，惊厥，甚至出现脱水，酸中毒，呼吸或循环衰竭。

Main manifestations: The axillary temperature exceeds 39℃(or

41 ℃ in severe cases). The high fever is accompanied by delirium, coma, or convulsions, or even with dehydration, acidosis, respiratory failure or circulatory failure in severe cases.

5.3.2 治疗
5.3.2 Treatment

处方：大椎、合谷(双)、风池(双)、曲池(双)或十宣。

针用泻法不留针，十宣放血。

神昏谵语加针人中、涌泉(双)、神门；斑疹隐隐加针血海(双)、曲泽(双)，委中三棱针放血；惊厥抽风加针内关(双)、阳陵泉(双)、太冲(双)，严重时可取十二井穴点刺出血。

耳针：取肾上腺、神门、交感、耳尖穴。

强刺激留针30分钟，耳尖放血2～3滴。

Prescription: Dazhui (DU 14), bilateral Hegu (LI 4), bilateral Fengchi (GB 20), bilateral Quchi (LI 11) and Shixuan (EX-UE11).

Puncture the points with reducing method and no needle retaining. The Shixuan is punctured to cause bleeding.

Supplementary points:

Delirium and loss of consciousness: Puncture Renzhong (DU 26) Yongquan (KI 1) and Shenmen (HT 7).

Rashes: Bilateral Xuehai (SP 10), bilateral Quze (PC 3) and pricking to let bleeding in Weizhong (BL 40);

Convulsions: Bilateral Neiguan (PC 6), bilateral Yanglingquan (GB 34), bilateral Taichong (LR 3) or pricking puncture in 12 jing-(well) points to make bleed;

Auricular points: Adrenal, Shenmen, Sympathetic, Apex of the Ear. Apply intense stimulation and retain the needles for 30 minutes.

Prick the ear apex to make bleed (2—3 drops of blood).

5.4 溺水
5.4 Near-Drowning

5.4.1 辨证
5.4.1 Differentiation

主要表现:面色青紫,偶或有喘息数次,咽喉部有气过水声,瞳孔缩小,肌张力尚可,心音微弱,脉搏急促;溺水时间较长病情严重者,捞出时可见面色及皮肤苍白冰冷,呼吸停止,瞳孔散大,心音微弱,肌张力消失,脉微欲绝。

Main manifestations: Purplish face, occasional breathing, miosis, weak heart beats, rapid pulse. If the patient is submerged in the water for a longer period of times, he may have the pale and cold skin, no respiration, mydriasis, weak heart beats, muscle paralysis, extreme weak pulse and difficult to feel.

5.4.2 治疗
5.4.2 Treatment

处方:会阴、人中、中冲(双)、素髎。
Prescription: Huiyin(RN 1), Renzhong(DU 26). bilateral Zhongchong(PC 9) and Suliao(DU 25).

5.5 急性一氧化碳中毒
5.5 Acute Carbon Monoxide Poisoning

5.5.1 辨证
5.5.1 Differentiation

主要表现:中毒轻者感头痛欲裂,头胀头晕,耳鸣,眼花,心跳,乏力,恶心,呕吐,视力模糊;中毒严重者出现昏厥,抽搐,肌束颤动,呼吸急促,口唇粘膜呈樱桃红色,瞳孔扩大,脉搏促急,最后出现呼吸麻痹而死亡。

Main manifestations: In mild case, the patient may have severe headache, dizziness, tinitus, blurred vision, palpitation, lassitude, nausea, and vomiting. The fainting, convulsions, trembling muscle, respiratory distress, cherry lips, mydriasis and rapid pulse may be seen in severe cases. The patients may die of respiratory paralysis.

5.5.2 治疗
5.5.2 Treatment

处方:人中、涌泉、合谷、中冲。
针用强刺激;中冲刺血。
汗闭者加梅花针叩刺4~7颈椎,头痛、眼花者加叩刺前额区。

Prescription: Renzhong(DU 26), Yongquan(KI 1), Hegu(LI 4) and Zhongchong(PC 9).

Apply intense stimulation in the points and prick PC 9 for bloodletting.

5.6　高山反应
5.6　Altitude Stress

5.6.1　辨证
5.6.1　Differentiation

主要表现：初到高原地区或登山过程中，患者感头痛，心慌，胸闷，呼吸急促，颜面潮红，心跳加速，严重反应者可出现精神变态，视听障碍，血压升高，唇甲发绀，呼吸困难，心脏扩大，甚则出现心衰，昏迷。

Main manifestations: Newly settling in high altitude area or during the mountain climbing, the patient experiences the headache, palpitation, rapid and short breathing, pressing feeling in the chest and flushed complexion, and may have rapid heart beats. Trance, optical and audile disturbance, hypertension, purplish lips and nails, and difficulty of breathing, or even heart failure and coma, may be seen in severe cases.

5.6.2　治疗
5.6.2　Treatment

处方：内关(双)。

针用泻法，留针10～30分钟。

昏迷者加针人中、十宣刺血；头痛、头晕者可加百会、风池；血压升高者可加曲池、足三里；气短者可加天突、膻中、肺俞。

Prescription: Neiguan (PC 6) bilaterally.

Supplementary points:

Coma: Renzhong(DU 26), Shixuan (EX-UE11) are pricked for bloodletting;

Headache and dizziness: Baihui(DU 20) and Fengchi(GB 20);

Hypertension: Quchi(LI 11), and Zusanli(ST 36); and

Rapid and short breathing: Tiantu(RN 20), Tangzhong(RN 17) and Feishu(BL 13).

5.7 放射反应
5.7 Radioreaction

由于接受钴^{60}或用镭锭或用镭—钴^{60}以及深度X线体外照射等治疗而引起的不良反应。

This disorder includes the side effects of Cobalt-60 therapy, or Radium-Cobalt-60 therapy and the intense X-ray radiation.

5.7.1 辨证
5.7.1 Differentiation

主要表现:头痛,头晕,恶心,呕吐,乏力,厌食,失眠,腹胀,腹泻等,实验室检查表现有白细胞减少。

Main manifestation: Headache, dizziness, nausea, vomiting, lassitude, poor appetite, insomnia, abdominal fullness, diarrhoea, and leukopenia.

5.7.2 治疗
5.7.2 Treatment

处方:大椎、合谷、曲池、足三里。

针用平补平泻,留针 15~30 分钟;若有畏寒、肢冷等虚寒证者,可酌加灸法,针灸并用。

检查有白细胞减少者可加针大杼、脾俞、膈俞、肾俞、内关等;恶心呕吐、腹痛腹泻者可加针中脘、天枢、建里、内关、章门、气海;头痛、头晕、失眠者可加针太阳、上星、头维、百会、神门、三阴交。

Prescription: Dazhui(DU 14), Hegu(LI 4), Quchi(LI 11) and Zusanli(ST 36).

Apply even method in the points and retain the needles for 15—30 minutes. Apply moxibustion or both acupuncture and moxibustion in cases with deficient cold syndrome.

Supplementary points:

Leukopenia: Dazhu(BL 11), Pishu(BL 20), Geshu(BL 17), Shenshu(BL 23) and Neiguan(PC 6);

Nausea, vomiting, diarrhoea and abdominal pain: Zhongwan(RN 12), Tianshu(ST 25), Jianli(RN 11), Neiguan(PC 6), Zhangmen(LR 13) and Qihai(RN 6); and

Headache, dizziness and insomnia: Taiyang(EX-HN15), Shangxin(DU 22), Touwei(ST 8), Baihui(DU 20), Shenmen(HT 7) and Sanyinjiao(SP 9).

5.8 急性白血病
5.8 Acute Leukemia

5.8.1 辨证
5.8.1 Differentiation

主要表现:患者可见急性贫血,进行性加重,可有发热,衰竭,苍白,皮肤及粘膜出血,口腔及咽峡部有坏死性溃疡,齿龈肿胀或出血发炎等,有时可触及到肿大的肝、脾及淋巴结。

Main manifestations: Acute and progressive anemia, high fever, depletion, pale skin, subcutaneous and musocal bleeding, necrotized ulcers in mucosa of mouth cavity and isthmuis faccium, swelling gums, gums bleeding. Physical examination reveals enlargment of spleen, liver or lymph nodes.

5.8.2 治疗
5.8.2 Treatment

瘢痕灸法。
取大椎、膏盲俞、四花穴。
1次或分次施灸。

Prescription: Dazhui (DU 14), Gaohuang shu (BL 43), Sihuaxue (Four-flower points, bilateral Danshu, BL 19 and bilateral Geshu, BL 17).

Apply scarring moxibustion.

5.9 心绞痛
5.9 Angina Pectoris

5.9.1 辨证
5.9.1 Differentiation

主要表现:突然发作的胸骨下段后面或心前区钳夹样、压榨样剧痛,呈阵发性。常向左肩左臂放散,伴恐惧感,每次发作持续数秒至数分钟,持续时间极少超过15分钟。

Main manifestations: Sudden attacks of retrosternal constricting and oppressive pain or gripping pain. The pain commonly radiates to the left shoulder and left arm, accompanied with apprehension. The pain lasts several seconds to several minutes; but seldomly exceeds 15 minutes.

5.9.2 治疗
5.9.2 Treatment

处方:膻中、内关、心俞、厥阴俞、足三里。

针用泻法,留针20～30分钟,每3～5分钟行针一次。

痰喘气涌者加针肺俞、丰隆;五心烦热,颧红,咽干者加针太溪、三阴交;心血瘀阻,舌上瘀斑者,加针血海、膈俞;形寒肢冷,气短脉微者,加灸关元、气海;血压下降者,加针涌泉、合谷。

耳针:取内分泌、交感、神门和心、肺、气管、食道穴。

针用泻法:留针1小时,每10分钟捻转1次或埋针。

Prescription: Tangzhong (RN 17), Neiguan (PC 6), Xinshu (BL

15) Jueyinshu(BL 14) and Zusanli(ST 36).

Puncture the points with reducing method and retain the needles for 20—30 minutes. Manipulate the needles once every 3—5 minutes.

Supplementary points:

Distress in chest and profuse sputum: Feishu(BL 13) and Fenglong (ST 40);

Restlessness and hot sensation in palms, soles and in the chest, dry throat: Taixi(KI 3), Sanyinjiao(SP 9);

Heart blood stagnation: Xuehai(SP 10) and Geshu(BL 17);

Cold limbs and body, shortness of breathing and weak pulse: Apply moxibustion in Guanyuan(RN 4) and Qihai(RN 6); and

Hypotension: Yongquan(KI 1) and Hegu(LI 4).

Auricular points: Endocrine, Trachea or Esophagus.

Puncture the points with filiform needles and retain the needles for one hour. Twirle the needles once every 10 minutes or embed the needles in the points.

5.10 心肌梗塞
5.10 Myocardiac Infarction

5.10.1 辨证
5.10.1 Differentiation

主要表现：实然发生胸骨下段后面或心前区绞窄样剧痛，并可向左肩、左臂或上腹部放射；疼痛持续数小时，甚至1—2天以上，常伴有血压下降，恐惧不安，汗出肢冷，脉微欲绝，甚至恶心呕吐，多数病人在发病数小时后即伴有体温升高,少数在 24—48 小时后才上升,持续 1 周左右。

Main manifestations: Sudden attacks of severe retrosternal or precardial constricting and opressive pain. The pain may radiates to left shoulder, left arm or upper abdomen. The pain may last for several hours, or even for one to two days. The patients commonly have hypotension, apprehension, profuse cold sweating, extremely weak pulse and difficult to feel, or nausea and vomiting. Most of the patients have a fever several hours after the onset of the attack, while in some cases fever occour 24—48 hours after the onset of attack. The fever usually lasts about one week.

5.10.2 治疗
5.10.2 Treatment

处方:内关(双)、心俞(双)、膻中。

针用泻法:留针 15~30 分钟,每日 1~2 次。

前胸刺痛加针厥阴俞、膈俞;心律不齐加针神门、足三里;气短痰多加针肺俞、丰隆;血压下降加针涌泉、合谷,并灸关元、气海;心跳暂停加针间使、足三里。

Prescription: Neiguan (PC 6d), Xinshu (BL 15), and Tangzhong (RN 17). Puncture the points with reducing method. Retain the needles for 15—30 minutes. One or two treatments daily.

Supplementary points:

Precardial twinge: Jueyinshu (BL 14) and Geshu (BL 17);

Arrhythmia: Shenmen (HT 7), Zusanli (ST 36);

Distress in chest and profuse sputum: Feishu (BL 13) and Fenglong (ST 40);

Hypotension: Yongquan(KI 1) and Hegu(LI 4); and apply moxibustion in Guanyuan(RN 4) and Qihai(RN 6); and

Cardiac arrest: Puncture Jianshi(PC 5) and Zusanli(ST 36).

5.11 急性胆囊炎
5.11 Acute Cholecystitis

5.11.1 辨证
5.11.1 Differentiation

主要表现:右上腹或右肋阵发性绞痛,常向右肩及右肩胛放射,患者出现恶寒发热,脉搏加快,或见高热,胆囊区明显触痛。

Main manifestations: Paroxysmal colicky pain in upper right abdomen. The pain commonly radiates to right shoulder. The patients may have chills and fever, rapid pulse, or high fever, or prominent tenderness over the gallbladder region.

5.11.2 治疗
5.11.2 Treatment

处方:日月、期门、肝俞、胆俞、配内关、阳陵泉、太冲。

针用泻法,每5分钟行针1次,留30分钟。高热不退可加针合谷、曲池、大椎;恶心呕吐可加针足三里、中脘、丘墟。

Prescription: Riyue(GB 24), Qimen(LR 14), Ganshu(BL 18), Danshu(BL 19), Neiguan(PC 6), Yangligquan(GB 34) and Taichong(LR 3).

Puncture the points with reducing method and retain the needles for 30 minutes. Manipulate the needles once every five minutes.

Supplementary points:

Persistent high fever: Hegu(LI 4), Quchi(LI 11) and Dazhui(DU 14); and

Nausea and vomiting: Zusanli(ST 36), Zhongwan(RN 12) and Qiuxu(GB 40).

5.12 胆石症
5.12 Gallstone

5.12.1 辨证
5.12.1 Differentiation

主要表现:突然发生的右上腹或右胁下,阵发性绞痛,痛引右肩背部,并有反射性恶心呕吐,吐后疼痛不减;疼痛发生12小时后出现黄疸。

Main manifestations: Sudden paroxysmal colicky pain in right upper abdomen. The pain commonly radiates to right shoulder and back. The patients may have reflective nausea and vomiting. The pain is not relieved after vomiting. The jaundice usually occurs 12 hours after the onset of the pain.

5.12.2 治疗
5.12.2 Treatment

处方:右胆俞、日月、期门、中脘。

配穴:足三里、阳陵泉、丘墟、太冲。

针用泻法,留针30分钟,每3~5分钟行针1次,每日治疗1~2次。

并发绞痛、疼痛严重者可加针合谷;呕吐者可加针内关;出现高热者可加针曲池;有黄疸出现者可加针至阴。

耳针:取神门、交感、肝、胆胰区、十二指肠穴。耳反应敏感的耳穴2~3对,重刺激,留针30分钟,每日1~2次,平时自行用手按捏留针(压丸)处1~2分钟,每日3~5次。

Prescription:

Dominant Points: Right Danshu(BL 19), Riyue(GB 24), Qimen(LR 14) and Zhongwan(RN 12).

Supporting Points: Zusanli(ST 36), Yanglingquan(GB 34), Qiuxu(GB 40) and Taichong(LR 3).

Puncture the points with reducing method. Retain the needles for 30 minutes and manipulate the needles once every 3—5 minutes.

Supplementary points:

Colicky pain: Hegu(LI 4);

Vomiting: Neiguan(PC 6);

High fever: Quchi(LI 11); and

Jaundice: Zhiyin(BL 67).

Auricular points: Shenmen, Sympathetic, Liver, Gallbladder Pancreas and Duodenum.

Two to three points are used each time with intense stimulation.

Retain the needls for 30 minutes. One or two treatment daily. Or advise the patients to press the points 3—5 times daily, 1—2 minutes each time.

5.13 胆道蛔虫症
5.13 Biliary Ascariasis

5.13.1 辨证
5.13.1 Differentiation

主要表现:右上腹或剑突下钻顶样剧痛,阵发性,痛引右肩背,严重者弯腰屈膝、捧腹、肢冷汗出,但发作间歇期间不出现症状,一如常人。若有恶心呕吐或吐蛔者,对本病诊断有一定意义,部分病人可有黄疸。此病症多发于儿童和青壮年。

Main manifestations: Severe paroxysmal boring pain under the xiphoid process or in right upper abdomen with profuse cold sweating. The pain radiates to the right shoulder. During the intermission of attacks, the patients feel no symptoms. The nausea and vomiting, or vomiting the ascarides, are helpful in making a diagnosis. Jaundice may be seen in some cases. The disease is often seen in children, teenagers and young persons.

5.13.2 治疗
5.13.2 Treatment

处方:迎香透四白;中脘透梁门、天枢;胆囊穴、右胆俞、中脘、鸠尾。

上穴任选一组,针用泻法,留针20~30分钟。

有呕吐者可加针内关、足三里;蛔虫多者可加针关元、太冲以加强驱蛔作用。

耳针：取胆、肝、神门、交感、十二指肠穴。

针用强刺激法，留针 20～30 分钟。

Prescription: (1). Yingxiang (LI 20) penetrating through Sibai (ST 2);(2). Zhongwan (RN 12) penetrating through Liangmen (ST 21), Tianshu (ST 25);and (3)Right Danshu (BL 19), Zhongwan (RN 12) and Jiuwei (RN 15), Dalanshu (EX-LE6). Choose one group of points each time. Puncture the points with the reducing method. Retain the needles for 20-30 minutes.

Supplementary points:

Vomiting:Neiguan(PC 6d) and Zusanli(ST 36);

Vomiting ascarides:Guanyuan(RN 4) and Taichong(LR 3).

Auricular points: Gallbladder, Liver, Shenmen, Sympathetic Nerve and Duodenum points.

Puncture the points with intense stimulation and retain the needles for 20-30 minutes.

5.14 消化性溃疡急性穿孔
5.14 Acute Perforation of Peptic Ulcer Diseases

5.14.1 辨证
5.14.1 Differentiation

主要表现：突然发生上腹剧疼，持续加重，并逐渐波及全腹，变动体位时腹痛加剧；烦躁不安，血压下降，汗出，肢冷，脉搏急促等休克症状；腹式呼吸变浅（或消失），腹肌强直，压痛，反跳痛明显加剧。肝浊音界缩小或消失，肠鸣音减弱或消失，叩诊可出现腹腔内移动性浊音。

Main manifestations: Sudden attacks of severe pain in upper abdomen. The pain is persistent and progressive, and involves the whole abdomen gradually. The pain become worse in changing the body position. The patients may have the manifestations of shock such as, restlessness, hypotension, cold limbs and profuse sweating, and rapid pulse. Physical examination may reveal abdominal muscular tension, prominent tenderness, rebounding tenderness, shifiting dullness, diminution or disappearance of hepatic dullness.

5.14.2 治疗

5.14.2 Treatment

处方：足三里、中脘、梁门、天枢、内关。

针用泻法，留针1小时，每15分钟捻针1次，每日治疗3—4次，至症状缓解后可逐渐减少针刺次数。

Prescription: Zusanli (ST 36), Zhongwan (RN 12), Liangmen (ST 21) and Neiguan (PC 6).

Puncture the points with reducing method. Retain the needles for one hour and manipulate the needles once every 15 minutes. Three to four treatments daily.

5.15 急性幽门梗阻
5.15 Acute Pylorochesis

5.15.1 辨证
5.15.1 Differentiation

主要表现:上腹胀痛,呕吐,呕吐物为胃酸及食物残渣,伴饭后30分钟左右腹胀,反胃,吐食,嗳气,吞酸等。

Main manifestations: Upper abdominal pain, vomiting the gastric juice and residue of foods. The patients commonly have abdominal fullness, regurgitation, belching or vomiting about 30 minutes after meal.

5.15.2 治疗
5.15.2 Treatment

处方:内关、中脘、足三里。
配穴:脾俞、胃俞、梁门、气海、曲池、合谷、金津玉液。
针用泻法,按内关、中脘、足三里的顺序针刺,留针15～30分钟,每3～5分钟行针一次。适当选用配穴1－2对以配合治疗。
受寒引起者可加灸气海、中脘、足三里穴。

Prescription

Dominant Points: Neiguan(PC 6), Zhongwan (RN 12) and Zusanli(ST 36).

Supportive Points: Pishu(BL 20), Weishu(BL 21), Lianmen(ST 21), Qihai(RN 6), Quchi(LI 11), Hegu(LI 4) and Jinjinyuyi(EX-HN12,13).

Puncture the dominant points with reducing method in an order from Neiguan, Zhongwan, to Zusanli. Retain the needles for 15—30 minutes and manipulate the needles once every 3—5 minutes. One to two supportive points could be selected together with the dominant points. For cases caused by cold evil invasion, combining the acupuncture with moxibustion in Qihai(RN 6), Zhongwan(RN 12) and Zusanli (ST 36).

5.16 急性肠梗阻
5.16 Acute Intestinal Obstruction

5.16.1 辨证
5.16.1 Differentiation

主要表现:突然发作的阵发性腹痛,呕吐剧烈,常吐出胆汁、粪水。腹胀,可见肠型、无排便、无排气,肠鸣音阵发性亢进,有气过水声者为单纯机械性梗阻。腹痛呕吐持续加剧,则出现腹肌紧张,触痛明显,肠鸣反而渐弱,血压下降,汗出肢冷,气促脉疾者为绞窄性梗阻。若腹胀明显,而腹痛、呕吐不明显及肠鸣反减弱,无排气者,可能为麻痹性梗阻。

Main manifestations: Sudden attacks of paroxysmal abdominal pain, severe vomiting with biliary juice or feces. In cases of simple intestinal obstruction, the patient may have abdominal fullness, constipation and no gas passing. And physical examination reveals visible peristalsis, paroxysmal hyperactivity of bowel sound and sound of air passing water. In cases of strangulated intestinal obstruction, the patient may have persistent and severe vomiting and abdominal pain. Physical examination reveals tenderness and abdominal muscular tension, diminution of bowel sound, hypotension, cold limbs and profuse sweating, rapid breathing and rapid pulse. The patients with paralytic intestinal obstruction may have prominent fullness of abdomen, diminution of bowel sound, no gas passing, and have only mild abdominal pain and vomiting.

5.16.2 治疗

5.16.2 Treatment

处方：足三里、内庭、天枢、中脘、合谷、大横。

针用泻法、强刺激，留针30—60分钟，每5分钟行针1次，每4—6小时治疗1次。

虚寒者可用艾条灸气海、关元、足三里，发热可加针曲池；呕吐可加针内关、上脘；腹痛可加针内关、章门；腹胀或小腹痛可加针关元、气海，针用泻法并灸。

Prescription: Zusanli (ST 36), Neiting (ST 44) and Daheng (SP 15). Puncture the points with reducing method. Apply the intense stimulation and retain the needles for 30—60 minutes. Manipulate the needles once every five minutes. One treatment every 4—6 hours.

Supplementary points:

Case with deficient cold syndrome: apply moxibustion in Qihai (RN 6), Guanyuan (RN 4) and Zusanli (ST 36)

Fever: Quchi (LI 11)

Vomiting: Neiguan (PC 6) and Shangwan (RN 13)

Abdominal pain: Neiguan (PC 6) and Zhangmen (LR 13)

Abdominal fullness and lower abdominal pain: Apply acupuncture and moxibustion in Guanyuan(RN 4) and Qihai(RN 6).

5.17 急性胰腺炎
5.17 Acute Pancreatitis

5.17.1 辨证
5.17.1 Differentiation

主要表现：忽然发生上腹正中或偏左剧烈疼痛，如刀割、灼痛，常向左肋、左肩、左背放散，伴恶心呕吐，腹胀便秘，兼见发热(38～39℃)，畏寒，甚至有血压下降、四肢厥冷、脉快而弱等休克现象。

Main manifestations: Sudden attacks of middle upper or left upper abdominal lancinating or burning pain. The pain radiates to the left shoulder, back and left hypochondriac region, and is accompanied with nausea, vomiting, abdominal fullness and constipation, or chills and fever (38—39 ℃). The manifestations of shock such as, cold limbs, rapid and weak pulse, may be seen in severe cases.

5.17.2 治疗
5.17.2 Treatment

处方：上脘、中脘、足三里、下巨虚、地机。

针用泻法，强刺激，留针60～90分钟，每5～10分钟行针1次，每日治疗2～3次。

呕吐者可加针内关；发热者可加针合谷；黄疸者可加针阳陵泉；腹痛者可加针梁门、章门或阿是穴(胰腺部位压痛点)深刺，及脾俞、胃俞、内庭、日月、期门等。

耳针：取胆、胰、交感、神门穴。

强刺激，留针 1 小时，每日 2~3 次，亦可用埋针疗法。

Prescription: Shangwan(RN 13), Zhongwan(RN 12), Zusanli(ST 36), Xiajuxu(ST 39) and Diji(SP 8).

Puncture the points with the reducing method and intense stimulation. Manipulate the needles once every 5—10 minutes. Two to three treatments daily.

Supplementary points:

Vomiting: Neiguan(PC 6);

Fever: Hegu(LI 4);

Jaundice: Yanglingquan(GB 34);

Abdominal pain: Liangmen(ST 21), Zhangmen(LR 13), or puncture deeply in Ashi point (abdominal tenderness point around pancreas); or Pishu(BL 20), Weishu(BL 21), Neiting(ST 44), Riyue(GB 24) and Qimen(LR 14), etc.

Auricular points: Gallbladder, Pancreas, Sympathetic Nerve and Shenmen.

Puncture the points with intense stimulation and retain the needles for one hour. Two to three treatments daily. Or apply needle embeding.

5.18 急性阑尾炎
5.18 Acute Appendicitis

5.18.1 辨证
5.18.1 Differentiation

主要表现:突然发生腹痛,初起于脐周或上腹,数小时后渐转移至右下腹。腹痛为持续性或阵发性,兼见恶心、呕吐、便秘或腹泻和食欲不振。体温正常或略高,但很少超过 39℃。若骤然体温上升、高热、寒战、脉搏加快,常提示穿孔;若疼痛骤然自止,也提示穿孔或形成坏死之可能。

Main manifestations: Sudden abdominal pain. At first the pain is around the umbilicus, or in upper abdomen, then moves to right lower abdomen gradually. The pain is persistent or paroxysmal, and is accompanied with nausea, vomiting, constipation or diarrhoea, and poor appetite. Patients have normal temperature or mild fever (less than 39 ℃). A sudden rising temperature, chills and high fever, and rapid pulse commonly indicate the appendical perforation. A sudden alleviation of pain without treatment possibly indicates the appendical perforation or necrosis.

5.18.2 治疗
5.18.2 Treatment

处方:足三里、阑尾穴、下巨虚、阿是穴(右下腹压痛点)。

针用泻法,留针 30—60 分钟,每 5~10 分钟行针 1 次,每日治疗 2～3 次。

恶心呕吐者可加针内关、上脘、中脘；发热者可加针合谷、曲池；腹痛便秘者，可加针中脘、天枢。

灸法：用艾炷（枣核大）或艾卷（回旋灸），灸气海、阿是穴（压痛点）和阑尾穴，每穴 5～10 分钟。

耳针：取神门、交感、阑尾穴或大小肠之间敏感点。强刺激，留针 60 分钟，每日 1—2 次。

Prescription: Zusanli (ST 36), Lanweixue (EX-33), Xiajuxu (ST 39) and Ashi point (Tenderness points in lower right abdomen).

Puncture the points with reducing method and retain the needles for 30 — 60 minutes. The needled are manipulated once every 5 — 10 minutes. Two to three treatments daily.

Supplementary points:

Nausea and vomiting: Neiguan (PC 6), Shangwan (RN 13) and Zhongwan (RN 12);

Fever: Hegu (LI 4) and Quchi (LI 11);

Abdominal pain and constipation: Zhongwan (RN 12), Tianshu (ST 25), and moxibustion in Qihai (RN 6) and Lanweixue (EX-33).

Auricular points: Shenmen, Sympathetic Nerve, Appendices, or postive point between the points small intestine and large intestine.

Puncture the points with intense stimulation and retain the needles for 60 minutes. One to two treatments daily.

5.19 肾绞痛
5.19 Renal Colic

5.19.1 辨证
5.19.1 Differentiation

主要表现:突然发生阵发性刀割样剧烈疼痛,自肾区沿输尿管向阴部及股内侧放射,疼痛发作可持续几分钟或几十分钟以至几小时;兼见面色苍白,出冷汗,恶心呕吐,脉细数等,甚则昏倒或休克;有肾区叩击痛、肋脊角压痛。

Main manifestations: Sudden attacks of paroxysmal lancinating pain. The pain is over renal region and radiates to the external genitalia and medial aspect of the thigh. The pain, lasting for several minutes or several hours, is accompanied with pale complexion, cold sweating, nausea, vomiting, rapid and thready pulse. Shock may be seen in severe cases. Physical examination reverals percussion tenderness over the kidney region and tenderness in costovertebral angle.

5.19.2 治疗
5.19.2 Treatment

处方:肾俞、膀胱俞、京门、三阴交。

配穴:关元、中极、水道、照海、足三里、腹结。

针主穴后,根据绞痛部位适当配合选用1~2个配穴,针用泻法,留针30分钟。

耳针:肾、输尿管、皮质下、交感穴或耳壳敏感点。

强刺激,留针15~30分钟,每日1~2次。亦可埋针、压丸。

Dominant Points: Shenshu(BL 23), Pangguangshu(BL 28), Jinmen(BL 63) and Sanyinjiao(SP 6).

Supplementary Points: Guanyuan (RN 4), Zhongji (RN 3), Shuidao(ST 38), Zhaohai(KI 6), Zusanli(ST 36) and Fujie(SP 14).

Puncture the dominant points and 1—2 supplementary points with reducing method. Retain the needles for 30 minutes.

Auricular points: Kindney, Ureter, Subcortex and Sympathetic Nerve.

Puncture the points with the intense stimulation and retain the needles for 15—30 minutes. One to two treatments daily.

Needle-embeding and point-pressing are also advisable.

5.20 滞产
5.20 Prolonged Labor

5.20.1 辨证
5.20.1 Differentiation

主要表现:足月正常产妇产程已发动后,出现子宫阵缩乏力、间歇延长,产妇虚脱、衰竭,胎儿宫内窘迫状态,而第1产程已超过24小时者。

Main manifestations: Prolonged labor, inertia of uterus, prolonged intermittence of uterine contraction, collapse, depletion, fetal suffocation and the first stage of labor exceeding 24 hours.

5.20.2 治疗
5.20.2 Treatment

处方:合谷、三阴交、太冲、昆仑、至阴、秩边。

补合谷,泻三阴交,灸至阴;其它穴位,针用泻法,留针20~60分钟,间歇行针,至分娩为止。

耳针:取子宫、神门、交感、皮质下、肾、腰椎穴。

针用强刺激。

Prescription: Hegu (LI 4), Sanyinjiao (SP 9), Taichong (LR 3), Kunlun (BL 60), Zhiyin (BL 67) and Zhibian (BL 54).

Apply reinforcing method in Hegu (LI 4), reducing method in Sanyinjiao (SP 9) and moxibustion in Zhiyin (BL 67). Puncture the other points with reducing method. Retain each needle for 20—60 minutes. After the insertion of needles, the needles are manipulated one after another till the end of the parturition.

Auricular points: Uterus, Shenmen, Sympathetic Nerve, Subcortex, Kidney and lumbar Vertedra.

Puncture the points with intense stimulation.

5.21 新生儿窒息
5.21 Asphyxia Neonatorum

5.21.1 辨证
5.21.1 Differentiation

主要表现:轻度(青紫窒息):胎儿皮肤呈青紫或紫红色,口鼻周围呈灰色,偶有喘息 1-2 次,喉部有气过水声,瞳孔缩小,脉搏快而有力,肌张力好;重度(苍白窒息):皮肤厥冷,苍白或灰蜡色,呼吸停止,瞳孔散大,脉搏微弱甚则触不到,肌张力消失,心跳微弱。

Main manifestations: In mild asphyxia neonatorum, the patients may have cyanosis or purple skin, grey color in the region around the nose and lips, occasional breathing, miosis, rapid and forceful pulse, and fairly good muscular tension. The patients with severe asphyxia neoratorum may have cold and grey skin, no respiration, mydriasis, weak pulse and difficult to feel, disapperance of muscular tension, and very weak heart beats.

5.21.2 治疗
5.21.2 Treatment

处方:人中、素髎、十宣、百会。

针用泻法:留针 15~30 分钟,间歇行针。十宣用急刺法,不留针;百会用艾卷灸,直至啼哭或呼吸恢复为止。

Prescription: Renzhong (DU 26), Suliao (DU 25), Shixuan (EX-UE11) and Baihui (DU 20).

Puncture the DU 25 and DU 26 with reducing method and retain the needles for 15-30 minutes. Apply pricking puncture in Shixuan (EX-UE11) without needle-retaining. Apply moxibustion in Baihui (DU 20) till the appearance of crying or recovery of respiration.

5.22 急性湿疹
5.22 Acute Eczema

5.22.1 辨证
5.22.1 Differentiation

主要表现:关节屈侧多发,先有皮肤潮红,继而出现粟米大小之皮疹、渗液、糜烂,奇痒难忍,有烧灼或针刺感,结痂脱落后,色素沉着,此症常突然起病,呈对称性。

Main manifestations: It commonly occours in the flective side of joints and is manifestated as redish skin, erythema, vesiculation, weeping and severe itching with burning or pricking sensation. Pigmentation occours after scar is off. Its onset is sudden and has symmetric skin involvements.

5.22.2 治疗
5.22.2 Treatment

处方:大椎、曲池、三阴交、神门、血海、足三里、合谷。
针用泻法,留针15~30分钟,每日行针1~2次。

Prescription: Dazhui(DU 14), Quchi(LI 11), Sanyinjiao(SP 9), Shenmen(HT 7), Xuehai(SP 10), Zusanli(ST 36) and Hegu(LI 4). Puncture the points with reducing method and retain the needles for 15—30 minutes. One to two treatments daily.

5.23 破伤风
5.23 Tetanus

5.23.1 辨证
5.23.1 Differentiation

主要表现:发热,畏寒,头痛,乏力,咀嚼困难,烦躁不安,伤口掣痛,小儿易惊;严重者出现牙关紧闭,苦笑面容,四肢抽搐,全身痉挛,角弓反张,发作频繁,在声、光、搬动或用指轻弹面颊即可诱发抽搐。病人因喉头痉挛可引起窒息,面色苍白,口唇绀紫,呼吸极度困难,甚则衰竭。

Main manifestations: The mild cases may have chills and fever, headache, lassitude, difficult to chew, restlessness, pain in wound, and easy to fright in infantile. Frequent clenched jaws, facial muscle spasm, convulsions, generalized musclar spasm, and opisthotonus may been seen in severe cases. And the convulsions may be induced by the stimulation of sound, light, and by moving the patients, or slightly fingering on the cheek of patients. The suffocation due to laryngismus may develop; and the patients may have pale complexion, cyanosis of lips, respiratory distress and even depletion.

5.23.2 治疗
5.23.2 Treatment

处方:人中、风池、大椎、合谷、内关、太冲、后溪。
针用泻法,留针10~20分钟,间歇行针,每日1~3次。

高热者可加针风府、曲池；角弓反张者可加针至阳、筋缩；四肢抽搐者可加针曲池、阳陵泉；牙关紧闭者可加针颊车、翳风。

耳针：取皮质下、心、神门、枕、脑点等穴。

强刺激，留针1~2小时，每日1~3次。

Prescription: Renzhong(DU 26), Fengchi(GB 20), Dazhui(DU 14), Hegu(LI 4), Meiguan(PC 6), Taichong(LR 3) and Taixi(KI 3). Puncture the points with reducing method. One to three treatments daily.

Supplementary points:

High fever: Fengfu(DU 16) and Jinsuo(DU 8);

Gererlized convulsions: Quchi(LI 11) and Yanglingquan(GB 34); and

Clenched jaws: Jiache(ST 6) and Yifeng(SJ 17).

Auricular points: Subcortex, Shenmen, Occiput, Brain etc.

Puncture the points with intense stimulation and retain the needles for 1—2 hours. One to three treatments daily.

5.24 急性睾丸炎及附睾炎
5.24 Acute Testitis and Epididymo-orchitis

5.24.1 辨证
5.24.1 Differentiation

主要表现：患者突然出现睾丸或附睾肿胀、剧烈胀痛并牵引少腹及腹股沟部坠胀疼痛；阴囊皮肤紧张、红肿，伴有发热、恶寒等全身症状。

Main manifestations: Sudden testicular and orchiepidymal swelling, severe pain in scrotum, radiating to the lower abdomen, bearing-down pain in groin, red and tensive scrotal skin, swelling scrotum, chills and fever.

5.24.2 治疗
5.24.2 Treatment

处方：气海、关元、归来、三阴交、曲骨、气冲。
配穴：太冲、行间、大敦、中封、曲泉、阴陵泉、阳陵泉、合谷。
每次取主穴2~4个，配穴1~2个，针用泻法，留针15~30分钟，每日1~2次；虚寒患者可针后加灸。

Prescription

Dominant points: Qihai (RN 6), Guanyuan (RN 4), Guilai (ST 29), Sanyinjiao (SP 9), Qugu (RN 2) and Qichong (ST 30).

Supplementary points: Taichong (LR 3), Xingjian (LR 2), Dadun (LR 1), Zhongfeng (LR 4), Ququan (LR 8), Yinlingquan (SP 9), Yanglingquan (GB 34) and Hegu (LI 4).

Two to four dominant points and one to two supplementary points are used together in each treatment. Puncture the points with reducing method and retain the needles for 15 — 30 minutes. One to two treatments daily.

Apply moxibustion after acupuncture for cases of deficient cold syndrome.

5.25 食物中毒
5.25 Food Poisoning

5.25.1 辨证
5.25.1 Differentiation

主要表现:曾食用含有毒素或被细菌污染的食物,患者出现恶心,呕吐,腹痛,腹泻水样便等症状。兼见口唇干燥,皮肤弹性消失,目陷睛迷,血压下降,脉细弱,严重者出现休克而死亡。此症常集体发病。

Main manifestations: History of intaking foods contaminated by bacteria or toxin, nausea, vomiting, abdominal pain, diarrhoea with watery stools, accompanied with dry lips and skin, depressive eyes and blurred vision, hypotension, weak and thready pulse, and shock in severe cases.

5.25.2 治疗
5.25.2 Treatment

处方:中脘、天枢、足三里、关元。

针用强刺激,留针15~30分钟,每5分钟行针1次。

呕吐者可加针内关、尺泽及金津玉液或委中刺血;四肢厥逆冰冷,血压降低者可加针人中,灸神阙(隔盐);转筋、抽搐者可加针承山、阳陵泉,昏迷者可加针人中、中冲(刺血)、涌泉(刺血)。

Prescription: Zhongwam (RN 12), Tianshu (ST 21), Zusanli (ST 36) and Guanyuan (RN 4).

Puncture the points with the intense stimulation and retain the needles for 15—30 minutes.

Supplementary points:

Vomiting: Puncture Neiguan(PC 6), Chize(LU 5); Pricking Jinjin and Yuyi (EX-HN12 and EX-HN13) and Weizhong(BL 40) for blood-letting;

Cold limbs and hypotension: Puncture Renzhong(DU 26) and applying moxibustion in Shenque(RN 8) with partition of salt;

Muscular spasm or convulsions: Puncture Chenshan(BL 57) and Yanglingquan(GB 34); and

Loss of consciousness: Puncture Renzhong (DU 26), pricking Zhongchong(PC 9) and Yongquan(KI 1) for blood-letting.

5.26 输液反应
5.26 Anaphylatic Reaction in Transfusion

5.26.1 辨证
5.26.1 Differentiation

主要表现：患者常于输液后15～60分钟内突然出现寒战，高热，恶心，呕吐，皮肤潮红或荨麻疹；严重者可出现全身皮疹，呼吸困难，谵妄，昏迷，血压下降，二便失禁，甚至休克而死亡。

Main manifestations: The reaction commonly occurs 15—60 minutes after transfusion. The clinical manifestations include chills and fever, nausea, vomiting, redish skin or urticaria. Generalized rashes, respiratory distress, delirium, coma, hypotension and incontinence, or even shock, may be seen in severe cases.

5.26.2 治疗
5.26.2 Treatment

处方:合谷、曲池、关元、足三里。
灸关元,余穴强刺激捻针1~2分钟,留针15~30分钟。
耳针:取肾上腺。
埋针1~4小时。

Prescription: Hegu(LI 4), Quchi(LI 11), Guanyuan(RN 4) and Zusanli(ST 36).

Apply moxibustion in RN 4 and intense acupuncture stimulation in other points for 1—2 minutes. Retain the needles for 15—30 minutes.

Auricular points: Adrenal.

Apply needle-embeding in the point for 1—4 hours.

5.27 青霉素过敏反应
5.27 Anaphylatic Reaction to Penicillins

5.27.1 辨证
5.27.1 Differentiation

主要表现:患者在接触青霉素后,出现皮肤过敏反应,如荨麻疹、多形性红斑及接触性皮炎;重症则多在应用青霉素(皮试、外用、注射)5分钟左右或半小时内突然发生皮肤瘙痒、四肢发麻,继而胸闷、气紧、青紫、头晕、心慌、面色苍白、四肢麻木、恶心、呕吐或腹泻、自汗出、血压下降,甚则昏迷、抽搐、二便失禁。

Main manifestations: The reaction occours after exposure to penicillins, including skin reaction such as, urticaria, multiple erythema and contact dermatitis. In severe cases, the reaction, commonly occourring about five minutes after exposure to the penicillins, includes itching skin and numbness of limbs at first, then development to respiratory distress, cynarosis, dizziness, palpitation, pale complexion, nausea, vomiting, diarrhoea, profuse sweating, hypotension, and even coma, convulsions and incontinence.

5.27.2 治疗
5.27.2 Treatment

处方:人中、内关、曲池、血海、足三里、合谷、三阴交。
除人中外,余穴均取双侧。针用泻法。

Prescription: Renzhong(DU 26), Neiguan(PC 6), Quchi(LI 11), Xuehai(SP 10), Zusanli(ST 36), Hegu(LI 4) and Sanyinjiao(SP 9).

All the points, except the Renzhong(DU 26), are selected bilaterally. All the points are punctured with reducing method.

第六章 常用针灸处方
CHAPTER SIX COMMONLY-USED PRESCRIPTIONS OF ACUPUNCTURE AND MOXIBUSTION

6.1 闪腰类方
6.1 Prescriptions for Lumbago

6.1.1 闪腰一方
6.1.1 Prescription for Lumbago I

〔组成〕 人中。
Point:Renzhong(DU 26).
〔来源〕 彭静山教授经验方。
Source:Experience of Prof. Peng Jingshan.
〔功效〕 利腰通督止痛。
Action:Activating the circulation of blood and Qi in Du meridian, relieving the low back pain.
〔主治〕 腰部扭伤正中痛。
Indication:Lambago due to strain, pain in the middle region of low back.

〔用法〕 毫针泻法。
Application:Apply reducing method with filiform needle.

6.1.2 闪腰二方
6.1.2 Prescription for Lumbago II

〔组成〕 眼针膀胱区、肾区。
Points:Eye acupuncture:Urinary bladder and Kidney areas. (See Part one Chapter 4).

〔来源〕 作者经验方。
Source:Experience of authors.

〔功效〕 调经活血通络。
Action:Regulating and activating the blood circulation in collaterals.

〔主治〕 腰扭伤痛。
Indication:Lambago caused by strain.

〔用法〕 毫针刮针泻法。
Application:Apply reducing method by scrapping a filiform needle.

6.1.3 闪腰三方
6.1.3 Prescription for Lumbago III

〔组成〕 委中、腰部阿是。
Points:Weizhong (BL 40), Ashi points.

〔来源〕《医学正传》。
Source:Yi Xue Zhen Zhuan (Orthodox Medical Record).

〔功效〕 活血祛瘀止痛。
Action:Activating the blood circulation, removing the blood stasis and relieving pain.

〔主治〕 腰痛曲不能伸。
Indication: Low back pain, difficult to stretch.
〔用法〕 三棱针点刺出血。
Application: Apply spot pricking method for bloodletting with three-edged needle.

6.1.4 闪腰四方
6.1.4 Prescription for Lumbago IV

〔组成〕 腰痛点。
Point: Yaotongdian (EX-UE 7).
〔来源〕 朱振华《手针新疗法》。
Source: Shou Zhen Xin Liao Fa (New Therapeutic Technique of Hand Acupuncture).
〔功效〕 止腰痛。
Action: Relieving pain.
〔主治〕 腰扭伤两侧痛。
Indication: Low back pain due to strain, pain in the region beside the middle line of back.
〔用法〕 毫针泻法。
Application: Apply reducing method with filiform needle.

6.1.5 闪腰五方
6.1.5 Prescription for Lumbago V

〔组成〕 阿是、脾俞、膀胱俞。
Points: Ashi points, Pishu (BL 20), Pangguangshu (BL 28).
〔来源〕 司徒铃经验方。
Source: Prof. Situ Ling's Experience.

〔功效〕 祛湿活血通络。

Action: Dispelling the dampness, activating blood circulation and dredging the collaterals.

〔主治〕 腰扭伤伴湿困者。

Indication: Lower back pain due to strain accompanied by the manifestations of damp syndrome.

〔用法〕 挑治。

Application: Apply pricking therapy.

6.1.6 闪腰六方
6.1.6 Prescription for Lumbago VI

〔组成〕 环跳。

Point: Huantiao(GB 30).

〔来源〕《灸法秘传》。

Source: Jiufa Mi Chuan(Secrete Record of Moxibustion Therapy).

〔功效〕 通经络。

Action: Activating blood circulation in collaterals.

〔主治〕 腰痛,负重损伤不能转侧。

Indication: Lumbago caused by overloading, impairment in turning movement.

〔用法〕 艾灸。

Application: Apply moxibustion.

6.1.7 闪腰七方
6.1.7 Prescription for Lumbago VII

〔组成〕 印堂。

Point: Yintang(EX-HN 3).

〔来源〕 张玉春《中国针灸》1984(2)。

Source: Zhang Yucun, 1984(2) Chinese Acupuncture and Moxibustion.

〔功效〕 通络止痛。

Action: Dredging collaterals and relieving pain.

〔主治〕 急性腰扭伤。

Indication: Acute strain of low back.

〔用法〕 毫针针刺配合自身腰部运动。

Application: Needle the point and advise the patient to turn his waist when acupuncture is done.

6.1.8 闪腰八方

6.1.8 Prescription for Lumbago Ⅷ

〔组成〕 手扭伤1(食指与中指掌骨间隙)、扭伤2(中指与无名指掌骨间隙)。

Points: point 1: in the middle point of fissure between phalanges of index and middle fingers.

point 2: the middle point of the fissure between phalanges of middle and ring fingers.

〔来源〕 金长禄《中国针灸》1991(3)。

Source: Jin Changlu 1991(3) Chinese Acupuncture and Moxibustion.

〔功效〕 行气活血止痛。

Action: Activating the circulation of Qi and blood, relieving pain.

〔主治〕 急性腰扭伤。

Indication: Acute strain of low back.

〔用法〕 毫针针刺。

Application: Apply reducing method with filiform needle.

6.1.9 闪腰九方
6.1.9 Prescription for Lumbago Ⅸ

〔组成〕 手三里旁5分压痛敏感点。
Point: point 0.5 cun beside Shousanli(LI 10).

〔来源〕 林敏华《中国针灸》1989(4)。
Source: Li Minghua 1989(4) Chinese Acupuncture and Moxibustion.

〔功效〕 利腰脊。
Action: Benefitting the vertebral colum in lumbar region.

〔主治〕 急性腰扭伤。
Indication: Acute strain in low back.

〔用法〕 毫针针刺。
Application: Apply reducing method with filiform needle.

6.1.10 闪腰十方
6.1.10 Prescription for Lumbago Ⅹ

〔组成〕 奇功穴（按患者拇指和小指间的距离，从两踝间沿胫骨前嵴向上量取并向外侧旁开0.5cm处。
Point: Qigong(point with miracullous effect; located along the tibia crest, a palm breadth above the connecting line between the internal and external malleoluses, then 0.5cm beside the tibia crest).

〔来源〕 李华同《河南中医》1989(1)。
Source: Li Huatong 1989(1) Henan Journal of TCM.

〔功效〕 活血利腰。
Action: Activating the blood circulation, benefiting lumbar region.

〔主治〕 急性腰扭伤痛。
Indication: Acute strain of low back.

〔用法〕 毫针针刺,取穴男左女右。
Application: Apply reducing method with filiform needle, needle the point in left side for the male, in right side for the female.

6.1.11 闪腰十一方
6.1.11 Prescription for Lumbago XI

〔组成〕 天柱.
Point: Tianzhu(BL 10).

〔来源〕 何周智《云南中医杂志》1984(1)。
Source: He Zhouzhi 1984(1) Yunnan Journal of TCM.

〔功效〕 活血通络。
Action: Activating the blood circulation.

〔主治〕 急性腰扭伤。
Indication: Acute lumbago due to strain of low back.

〔用法〕 毫针泻法。
Application: Apply reducing method with filiform needle.

6.1.12 闪腰十二方
6.1.12 Prescription for Lumbago XII

〔组成〕 后溪。
Point: Houxi(SI 3).

〔来源〕 刘沁仁《湖北中医杂志》1984(1)。
Source: Liu Qinren 1984(1) Hubai Journal of TCM.

〔功效〕 通督脉、舒筋活血、消肿止痛。
Action: Activating the circulation of blood and Qi in Du meridian,

resolving the swelling and relieving pain.

〔主治〕 急性腰扭伤。

Indication:Acute lumbago due to strain in low back.

〔用法〕 毫针泻法。

Application:Apply reducing method with filiform needle.

6.2 止喘即效方
6.2 Prescriptions for the Attack of Asthma

6.2.1 止喘一方
6.2.1 Prescription for the Attack of Asthma I

〔组成〕 肺俞(双)、天突。

Points:Feishu(BL 13)bilateral,Tiantu(RN 23).

〔来源〕 《世医得效方》。

Source: Siyi Dexiao Fang (Effective Prescriptions for Generations).

〔功效〕 宣肺平喘。

Action:Regulating the Qi movement in Lungs,lowering the adverse rising Qi.

〔主治〕 寒哮型哮喘急性发作。

Indication:Asthma attack classfied as cold type.

〔用法〕 悬灸或直接灸。

Application:Apply moxibustion with moxa sticks or direct moxibustion.

6.2.2 止喘二方
6.2.2 Prescription for the Attack of Asthma Ⅱ

〔组成〕 四关穴。
Points:Four-gate points(bilateral LI 4 and LR 3).

〔来源〕 作者经验方。
Source:Experience of authors.

〔功效〕 调气降逆。
Action:Regulating the circulation of Qi,lowering the adverse rising Qi.

〔主治〕 热哮喘发作胸闷、口苦者。
Indication:Attack of asthma with full sensation in the chest and bitter taste in mouth due to heat pathogenic factor.

〔用法〕 毫针泻法。
Application:Apply reducing method with filiform needle.

6.2.3 止喘三方
6.2.3 Prescription for the Attack of Asthma Ⅲ

〔组成〕 鱼际(双)。
Points:BilateralYuji(LU 10).

〔来源〕 刘泽光《中国针灸》1986(2)。
Source:Liu Zeguan 1986(2)Chinese Acupuncture and Moxibustion.

〔功效〕 止咳平喘。
Action:Relieving cough and soothing asthma.

〔主治〕 哮喘发作。
Indication:Attack of asthma.

〔用法〕 毫针泻法。

Application:Apply reducing method with filiform needle.

6.2.4 止喘四方
6.2.4 Prescription for the Attack of Asthma IV

〔组成〕 大椎、肺俞(双)、风门(双)。

Points:Dazhui(DU 14),Feishu(BL 13)bilateral,Fengmen(BL 12)bilateral.

〔来源〕 何健等《中医杂志》(英文版)1988(3)

Source:He Jian etc. 1988(3)Journal of TCM(English edition).

〔功效〕 祛寒温肺平喘。

Action:Dispelling cold and warming lungs,soothing asthma.

〔主治〕 单纯性哮喘发作。

Indication:Attack of asthma without the complication.

〔用法〕 温针法。

Application:Apply needling,with moxibustion.

6.2.5 止喘五方
6.2.5 Prescription for the Attack of Asthma V

〔组成〕 头针胸腔区。

Point:Scalp acupuncture:Thoracic Area.

〔来源〕 焦顺发经验。

Source:Jiao Sunfa's experience.

〔功效〕 宽胸平喘。

Action:Releasing the full sensation in the chest and soothing asthma.

〔主治〕 急性哮喘发作。

Indication: Acute attack of asthma.

〔用法〕 毫针泻法。

Application: Apply reducing method with filiform needle.

6.2.6 止喘六方
6.2.6 Prescription for the Attack of Asthma Ⅵ

〔组成〕 听会(双)。

Point: Bilateral Tinghui (GB 2).

〔来源〕 陈作霖教授经验。

Source: Experience of Prof. Cheng Zuoling.

〔功效〕 平喘降逆。

Action: Lowering the adverse rising Qi and soothing asthma.

〔主治〕 哮喘发作。

Indication: Attack of asthma.

〔用法〕 毫针泻法。

Application: Apply reducing method with filiform needle.

6.2.7 止喘七方
6.2.7 Prescription for the Attack of Asthma Ⅶ

〔组成〕 手针咳喘点。

Point: Specific point for cough and asthma in Hand Acupuncture.

〔来源〕 朱振华《手针新疗法》。

Source: Shou Zhen Xin Liao Fa (New Therapy of Hand Acupuncture).

〔功效〕 止咳平喘。

Action: Relieving cough and soothing asthma.

〔主治〕 急性哮喘。

Indication: Acute asthma.

〔用法〕 毫针泻法。

Application: Apply reducing method with filiform needle.

6.2.8 止喘八方
6.2.8 Prescription for the Attack of Asthma Ⅷ

〔组成〕 大椎、肺俞、神阙。

Points: Dazhui(DU 14), Feishu(BL 13), Shenjue(RN 8).

〔来源〕 《古今医统》。

Source: Gujin Yitong (General Medicine of Past amd Present).

〔功效〕 纳气平喘。

Action: Invigorating the Kidney, improving Qi grasping function of kidney, soothing asthma.

〔主治〕 短气而喘。

Indication: Asthma attack with shortness of breath.

〔用法〕 艾灸。

Application: Apply moxibustion.

6.3 坐骨神经痛类方
6.3 Prescription for Sciatica

6.3.1 坐骨一方
6.3.1 Prescription for Sciatica Ⅰ

〔组成〕 眼针膀胱区、下焦、胆区。

Points: Eye Acupuncture: Urinary Bladder area, Lower Burner area, Gallbladder area.

〔来源〕 符文彬《中国针灸》1992(1)。
Source: Fu Wenbin 1992(1) Chinese Acupuncture and Moxibustion.

〔功效〕 通络止痛。
Action: Dredging the collaterals and relieving pain.

〔主治〕 各种原因引起坐骨神经痛。
Indication: Sciatica due to various causes.

〔用法〕 毫针刺法。
Application: Apply filiform needl acupuncture.

6.3.2 坐骨二方
6.3.2 Prescription for Sciatica II

〔组成〕 委中。
Point: Weizhong (BL 40).

〔来源〕 《针灸资生经》。
Source: Zhenjiu Zisheng Jing (Classic of Curing People with Acupuncture and Moxibustion).

〔功效〕 活血通络止痛。
Action: Activating the blood circulation, dredging the collateral relieving pain.

〔主治〕 腰腿重痛。
Indication: Pain and heavy sensation in legs and low back.

〔用法〕 三棱针刺络。
Application: Apply spot pricking for blood-letting with three-edged needle.

6.3.3 坐骨三方
6.3.3 Prescription for Sciatica Ⅲ

〔组成〕 坐骨神经穴(手背,无名指,掌指关节尺侧缘)。
Point:Sciatica point, on the back of the hand, in the ulnar side of the metacarpophalangeal joint of ring finger.

〔来源〕 朱振华《手针新疗法》。
Source:Shou zhen Xin Liao Fa (New Therapy of Hand Acupuncture).

〔功效〕 调经止痛。
Action:Regulating the function of meridian and relieving pain.

〔主治〕 坐骨神经痛。
Indication:Sciatica.

〔用法〕 毫针泻法。
Application:Apply reducing method with filiform needle.

6.3.4 坐骨四方
6.3.4 Prescription for Sciatica Ⅳ

〔组成〕 后溪、环跳。
Points:Houxi(SI 3),Huantiao(GB 30).

〔来源〕 《百证赋》。
Source:Baizhen Fu (The Poems about the Acupuncture Treatment of Syndromes).

〔功效〕 祛风湿通络止痛。
Action:Dispelling wind and dampness, activating the circulation of blood and Qi, relieving pain.

〔主治〕 风湿型坐骨神经痛。

Indication: Sciatica differentiated as wind-dampness.

〔用法〕 毫针泻法,亦可温针。

Application: Apply reducing method with filiform needle or apply warming needling.

6.3.5 坐骨五方
6.3.5 Prescription for Sciatica V

〔组成〕 脾俞、膀胱俞。
Points: Pishu(BL 20), Pangguangshu(BL 28).
〔来源〕 司徒铃教授经验方。
Source: Experience of Prof. Situ Ling.
〔功效〕 祛湿通络。
Action: Dispelling dampness and dredging collaterals.
〔主治〕 坐骨神经痛。
Indication: Sciatica.
〔用法〕 寒湿者可灸,气滞血瘀者可挑治。
Application: Apply moxibustion for cold-dampness, and apply pricking therapy for blood stagnation.

6.3.6 坐骨六方
6.3.6 Prescription for Sciatica VI

〔组成〕 环跳、风市、阴陵泉、委中、承山、悬钟。
Points: Huantiao(GB 30), Fengshi(GB 31), Yinlingquan(SP 9), Weizhong(BL 40), Chengshan(BL 57), Xianzhong(GB 39).
〔来源〕 夏玉卿经验方。
Source: Experience of Xia Yuqin.
〔功效〕 祛寒止痛。

Action: Dispelling cold and relieving pain.

〔主治〕 寒湿型坐骨神经痛。

Indication: Sciatica differentiated as cold-dampness type.

〔用法〕 火针焠刺。

Application: Apply the burning needling.

6.4 膝痛类方
6.4 Prescription for Knee Joint Pain

6.4.1 膝痛一方
6.4.1 Prescription for Knee Joint Pain Ⅰ

〔组成〕 环跳、委中。

Points: Huantiao(GB 30), Weizhong(BL 40).

〔来源〕 《内经》。

Source: Neijing.

〔功效〕 祛风湿活血通络。

Action: Dispelling dampness and wind, dreging the collaterals.

〔主治〕 膝关节肥大,风湿引起膝关节痛。

Indication: Swollen and painful knee joints due to wind-dampness.

〔用法〕 先泻环跳,后委中刺络。

Application: Apply reducing method in (GB 30), then apply spot pricking in Weizhong(BL 40).

6.4.2 膝痛二方
6.4.2 Prescription for Knee Joint Pain II

〔组成〕 膝阳关、脾俞、膀胱俞、膝阿是。
Points: Qiyangguan (GB 33), Pishu (BL 20), Pangguangshu (BL 28), Ashi points around the knee joint.

〔来源〕 作者验方。
Source: Experience of authors.

〔功效〕 祛湿散寒,消肿止痛。
Action: Dispelling cold and dampness, eliminating swelling and relieving pain.

〔主治〕 风湿型或寒湿型关节肿痛。
Indication: Painful and swollen knee joint due to wind-cold or due to cold-dampness.

〔用法〕 火针点刺。
Application: Apply spot pricking with burning neede.

6.4.3 膝痛三方
6.4.3 Prescription for Knee Joint Pain III

〔组成〕 曲泉、历兑。
Points: Ququan (KI 8), Lidui (ST 45).

〔来源〕 《神灸经纶》。
Source: Shenjiu Jinglun (The Protocol of Miraculous Moxibustion).

〔功效〕 散寒舒筋。
Action: Dispelling cold and relaxing tendons.

〔主治〕 膝关节冷痛。

Indication:Pain and cold sensation in knee joint.
〔用法〕 艾灸。
Application:Apply moxibustion.

6.4.4 膝痛四方
6.4.4 Prescription for Knee Joint Pain Ⅳ

〔组成〕 大陵、人迎。
Points:Daling(PC 7),Renyin(ST 9).
〔来源〕 彭静山《针灸秘验》。
Source:Zhen Jiu Mi Yan (The Secret Experience in Aupuncture and Moxibustion).
〔功效〕 活血通络,止痛。
Action:Dredging collaterals and relieving pain.
〔主治〕 膝关节痛。
Indication:Knee joint pain.
〔用法〕 毫针针刺。
Application:Apply reducing method with filiform needle acupuncture.

6.4.5 膝痛五方
6.4.5 Prescription for Knee Joint Pain Ⅴ

〔组成〕 膝阳关、委中、阳陵泉、中脘、丰隆。
Points:Qiyangguan (GB 33), Weizhong (BL 40), Yanglingquan (GB 34), Zhongwan (RN 12), Fenglong (ST 40).
〔来源〕《针灸大成》。
Source:Zhenjiu Dacheng (Achievements in Acupuncture and Moxibustion).

〔功效〕 清热利湿通络。

Action: Eliminating heat and dampness, activating the circulation of blood, dredging the collaterals.

〔主治〕 两膝关节红肿痛。

Indication: Swelling, redness and pain of Knee joints.

〔用法〕 委中刺络放血,余穴用泻法。

Application: Apply spot pricking therapy in Weizhong(BL 40), reducing method in the others.

6.4.6 膝痛六方
6.4.6 Prescription for Knee Joint Pain Ⅵ

〔组成〕 阴陵泉、中脘。

Points: Yinglingquan(SP 9), Zhongwan(RN 12).

〔来源〕 《针灸集成》。

Source: Zhenjiu Jicheng (A Collection of Acupuncture and Moxibustion Works).

〔功效〕 祛痰湿通络。

Action: Eliminating the dampness and phlegm and dredging the collaterals.

〔主治〕 膝上肿痛,伸屈不行。

Indication: Swelling and painful knee joint with difficulty to stretch and flex.

〔用法〕 阴陵泉用艾灸,中脘毫针泻法。

Application: Apply moxibustion in Yinlingquan (SP 9), reducing method in Zhongwan(RN 12).

6.5 中风偏瘫类方
6.5 Prescription for Hemiplegia after Apoplexy

6.5.1 中风一方
6.5.1 Prescription for Hemiplegia after Apoplexy Ⅰ

〔组成〕 眼针上焦、下焦。
Points:Eye Acupuncture;Upper and Lower Burner.
〔来源〕 彭静山《眼针疗法》。
Source:Peng Jingshan. "Eye Acupuncture Therapy".
〔功效〕 通经纠偏。
Action:Dredging the meridians and rectifying the hemiplegia.
〔主治〕 中风偏瘫。
Indication:Hemiplegia.
〔用法〕 毫针横刺。
Application:Apply filiform needle acupuncture with transverse insertion.

6.5.2 中风二方
6.5.2 Prescription for Hemiplegia after Apoplexy Ⅱ

〔组成〕 风池、大椎、肩井、间使、曲池、足三里、百会。
Points:Fengchi(GB 20),Dazhui(DU 14),Jianjing(GB 21),Jianshi(PC 5),Quchi(LI 11),Zusanli(ST 36),Baihui(DU 20).
〔来源〕 《千金方》。
Source:Qianjin Fang (Valuable Prescriptions).

〔功效〕 祛风活血通络。
Action: Dispelling the wind and dredging the collaterals.

〔主治〕 中风半身不遂。
Indication: Hemiplegia after the apoplexy.

〔用法〕 除大椎、百会外,先针健侧后针患侧。
Application: Except the Dazhui(DU 14), points in healthy limbs are needled at first, then those in the affected limbs.

6.5.3 中风三方
6.5.3 Prescription for Hemiplegia after Apoplexy Ⅲ

〔组成〕 头针运动区、四关穴。
Points: Motor area in scalp acupuncture, four-gate points (bilateral LI 4, and LR 3).

〔来源〕 作者经验方。
Source: Experience of authors.

〔功效〕 平肝熄风,活血通络。
Action: Calming the liver to inhibit the endogenous wind, activating the blood circulation and dredging the collaterals.

〔主治〕 中风偏瘫伴高血压者。
Indication: Hemiplegia after apoplexy accompanied by hypertension.

〔用法〕 毫针泻法。
Application: Apply reducing method with filiform needle.

6.5.4 中风四方
6.5.4 Prescription for Hemiplegia after Apoplexy Ⅳ

〔组成〕 阳陵泉、曲池。

Points: Yanglingquan (GB 34), Quchi (LI 11).

〔来源〕《百证赋》。

Source: Baizhen Fu (The Poems About Acupuncture Treatment of the Syndromes).

〔功效〕 活血舒筋,调和营卫气血。

Action: Activating the circulation of blood and Qi, relaxing the tendons, regulating the function of Ying (Nutritive) energy and Wei (Defensive) energy, regulating blood and Qi circulation.

〔主治〕 中风半身不遂。

Indication: Hemiplegia after apoplexy.

〔用法〕 毫针针刺。

Application: Apply reducing method with filiform needle.

6.5.5 中风五方
6.5.5 Prescription for Hemiplegia after Apoplexy V

〔组成〕 申脉、少商、前顶、人中、膻中、合谷、哑门。

Points: Shenmai (BL 62), Shaoshan (LU 11), Qianding (DU 21), Renzhong (DU 26), Tangzhong (RN 17), Hegu (LI 4), Yamen (DU 15).

〔来源〕《针灸大全》。

Source: Zhenjiu Daquan (A Complete Works of Acupuncture and Moxibustion).

〔功效〕 通络开窍。

Action: Dredging collaterals and opening the orifice of speaking.

〔主治〕 中风不语。

Indication: Dysphasia due to apoplexy.

〔用法〕 毫针泻法。

Application: Apply reducing method with filiform needle.

6.5.6 中风六方
6.5.6 Prescription for Hemiplegia after Apoplexy Ⅵ

〔组成〕 金津、玉液、廉泉、风府。
Points: Jinjin (EX-HN 12), Yuyi (EX-HN 13), Lianquan (RN 23), Fengfu (DU 16).

〔来源〕 《针灸大成》。
Source: Zhenjiu Dacheng (Achievements of Acupuncture and Moxibustion).

〔功效〕 祛风通络,开窍利言。
Action: Dispelling the wind, dredging the collaterals and opening the orifice of speaking.

〔主治〕 中风,舌强难言。
Indication: Dysphasia and rigidity of tongue in apoplexy.

〔用法〕 金津、玉液用三棱针点刺出血,廉泉、风府毫针泻法。
Application: Apply spot pricking and blood-letting in EX-HN 12 and 13 with three-edged needle, reducing method in Lianquan (RN 23) and Fengfu (DU 16).

6.6 面瘫类方
6.6 Prescriptions for Peripheral Facial Paralysis

6.6.1 面瘫一方
6.6.1 Prescription for Peripheral Facial Paralysis I

〔组成〕 颊车、地仓。
Points:Jiache(ST 6),Dicang(ST 4).
〔来源〕 《百证赋》。
Source:Baizheng Fu (The Poems About the Acupuncture Treatment of the Syndromes).
〔功效〕 祛风通络。
Action:Dispelling the exterior wind and dredging the collaterals.
〔主治〕 口喎。
Indication:Deviation of mouth.
〔用法〕 毫针透刺。
Application:Apply penetrating needling technique between two points.

6.6.2 面瘫二方
6.6.2 Prescription for Peripheral Facial Paralysis II

〔组成〕 人中、承浆、颊车、地仓、合谷。
Points:Renzhong (DU 26), Chengjiang (RN 24), Jiache (ST 6). Dicang(ST 4),Hegu(LI 4),Zusanli(ST 36).
〔来源〕 司徒铃教授经验方。

Source: Experience of Prof. Situ Ling.

〔功效〕 调气活血通络。

Action: Regulating circulation of blood and Qi, dreging the collaterals.

〔主治〕 口眼㖞斜。

Indication: Facial paralysis.

〔用法〕 颊车透地仓,人中、承浆用泻法,合谷用补法,足三里、地仓用直接灸.

Application: Apply penetrating puncture from ST 6 to ST 4, apply reducing method in DU 26 and RN 24; apply reinforcing method in LI 4, and direct moxibustion in ST 36 and ST 4.

6.6.3 面瘫三方

6.6.3 Prescription for Peripheral Facial Paralysis Ⅲ

〔组成〕 四关、翳风、阳白、耳尖。

Points: Four-gate points (bilateral LI 4 and LR 3), Yifeng (SI 17), Yangbai (GB 14), apex of the ears.

〔来源〕 作者验方。

Source: The experience of authors.

〔功效〕 平肝熄风通络。

Action: Calming the liver to inhibit the endogenous wind, dredging the collaterals.

〔主治〕 肝风内动型面瘫。

Indication: Facial paralysis accompanied by the upward stirring of liver-wind.

〔用法〕 耳尖放血,余穴毫针泻法。

Application: Apply blood-letting at the apex of the ears, reducing method in the others with filiform needles.

6.6.4 面瘫四方
6.6.4 Prescription for Peripheral Facial Paralysis Ⅳ

〔组成〕 外耳道。
Points: External Audiatory Canal.

〔来源〕 《针灸大成》。
Source: Zhenjiu Dacheng (The Achievements of Acupuncture and Moxibustion).

〔功效〕 祛邪通经。
Action: Dispelling the pathogenic factors and dredging collaterals.

〔主治〕 面瘫。
Indication: Facial paralysis.

〔用法〕 以五寸长竹管,插入耳道内,外以面粉塞四周,竹管上头以艾灸。
Application: Insert a five-cun long fine bamboo pipe into external auditory canal, fill the space around the pipe with the mixture of water and flour, then apply indirect moxibustion at the top of the pipe.

6.6.5 面瘫五方
6.6.5 Prescription for Peripheral Facial Paralysis Ⅴ

〔组成〕 地仓、颊车、听会、大椎、阳白、胃俞。
Points: Dicang(ST 4), Jiache (ST 6), Tinghui(GB 2), Dazhui(DU 14), Yangbai(GB 14), Weishu(BL 21).

〔来源〕 作者验方。
Source: Experience of Authors.

〔功效〕 温经通络。

Action:Warming the meridians and dredging collaterals.

〔主治〕 面瘫面部松驰者。

Indication:Facial paralysis with flaccid facial muscle in affected side.

〔用法〕 火针点刺。

Application:Apply spot pricking with burning needle.

6.6.6 面瘫六方
6.6.6 Prescription for Peripheral Facial Paralysis Ⅵ

〔组成〕 阳白、下关、颊车、地仓、大椎。

Points:Yangbai(GB 14),Xiaguan (ST 7),Jiache(ST 6),Dicang (ST 4),Dazhui(DU 14).

〔来源〕 曲祖贻验方。

Source:Experience of Qu Zuyi.

〔功效〕 祛风通络。

Action:Dispelling wind and dredging the collaterals.

〔主治〕 周围性面神经麻痹。

Indication:Peripheral facial paralysis.

〔用法〕 按上述穴位顺序连续闪罐。

Application:Apply swift cupping in the points according to the order listed.

6.6.7 面瘫七方
6.6.7 Prescription for Peripheral Facial Paralysis Ⅶ

〔组成〕 承泣、地仓、人迎。

Points:Chengqi(ST 1),Dicang (ST 4),Renyin(ST 9).

〔来源〕 《儒门事亲》。

Source: Lumen Si qin (Prorequistite Knowledge for Physicians).

〔功效〕 疏散风寒。

Action: Dispelling the cold and wind.

〔主治〕 口眼㖞斜。

Indication: Facial paralysis.

〔用法〕 先灸承泣、地仓,无效灸人迎。

Application: Apply moxibustion in ST 1 and ST 4, if no response, do it in ST 9.

6.7 呃逆类方
6.7 Prescriptions for Hiccup

6.7.1 呃逆一方
6.7.1 Prescription for Hiccup I

〔组成〕 期门、膻中、中脘。

Points: Qimen (LR 14), Tangzhong (RN 17), Zhongwan (RN 12).

〔来源〕 《医学纲目》。

Source: Yixue Gan Mu (Compendium of Medicine).

〔功效〕 疏肝和胃,降气止呃。

Action: Dispersing the stagnated liver energy, regulating the function of stomach

〔主治〕 呃逆。

Indication: Hiccup.

〔用法〕 用灸法。

Application: Apply the moxibustion.

6.7.2 呃逆二方
6.7.2 Prescription for Hiccup Ⅱ

〔组成〕 公孙、内关。
Points:Gongsun(SP 4),Neiguan(PC 6).
〔来源〕 《针经指南》。
Source:Zhen Jing Zhi Nan (Direction of Acupuncture Classic).
〔功效〕 调气降逆。
Action:Regulating the function of the stomach, lowering the adverse rising energy.
〔主治〕 呃逆。
Indication:Hiccup.
〔用法〕 毫针泻法。
Application:Apply reducing method with filiform needle.

6.7.3 呃逆三方
6.7.3 Prescription for Hiccup Ⅲ

〔组成〕 扶突。
Point:Futu(LI 18).
〔来源〕 蒋幼光验方。
Source:Experience of Jiang Youguan.
〔功效〕 降气止呃。
Action:Regulating the function of the stomach, lowering the adverse rising energy.
〔主治〕 心肌梗塞、膈肌裂孔疝、食道癌术后、中风后遗症、慢性肾炎尿毒症等并发顽固性呃逆。
Indication:The refractory hiccup appearing in myocardial infarc-

tion, hiatal hernia of diaphragm, postoperative esophagus carcinoma, sequenlae of apoplexy and uremia in chronic nephritis.

〔用法〕 毫针针刺,针尖稍偏向后下方,深度 0.5~0.7 寸,并且要求针感为触电感。

Application: Apply filiform needle acupuncture, the direction of needling is slightly toward posterior inferior with a insertion depth of 0.5 to 0.7 cun. A shock-like sensation of acupuncture is required.

6.7.4 呃逆四方
6.7.4 Prescription for Hiccup Ⅳ

〔组成〕 中魁。
Point: Zhongkui(EX-UE 4).
〔来源〕 《玉龙经》。
Source: Yulong Jing (The Classic of Jade Dragon).
〔功效〕 降逆止呃。
Action: Lowering the adversely rising Qi and supressing hiccup.
〔主治〕 胃寒型呃逆。
Indication: Hiccup, cold type in the stomach.
〔用法〕 直接灸。
Application: Apply direct moxibustion.

6.7.5 呃逆五方
6.7.5 Prescription for Hiccup Ⅴ

〔组成〕 天突、中脘。
Points: Tiantu(RN 22), Zhongwan(RN 12).
〔来源〕 《针灸正宗》。
Source: Zhenjiu Zhenzong (The Orthodox of Acupuncture and

Moxibustion).

〔功效〕 和胃降逆。

Action: Regulating the function of the stomach, lowering the adversely rising Qi.

〔主治〕 呃逆。

Indication: Hiccup.

〔用法〕 泻天突,补中脘。

Application: Apply reducing method in RN 22 and reinforcing method in RN 12.

6.7.6 呃逆六方
6.7.6 Prescription for Hiccup Ⅵ

〔组成〕 四关、医风。

Points: Four-gate Points (Bilateral LI 4 and LR 3), Yifeng (SJ 17).

〔来源〕 作者经验方。

Source: Experience of authors.

〔功效〕 疏肝理气降逆。

Action: Dispersing the stagnated liver energy, regulating the function of stomach and lowering the adverse rising Qi.

〔主治〕 肝胃不和型呃逆。

Indication: Hiccup differentiated as the disharmony between the liver and stomach.

〔用法〕 毫针泻法。

Application: Apply reducing method with filiform needle.

6.8 胃痛类方
6.8 Prescriptions for Stomachache

6.8.1 胃痛一方
6.8.1 Prescription for Stomachache I

〔组成〕 眼针胃区、中焦。
Points: Eye acupuncture; Stomach and Middle Burner areas.
〔来源〕 作者经验方。
Source: Experience of Authors.
〔功效〕 解痉止痛。
Action: Releasing the spasm and relieving pain.
〔主治〕 急性胃脘痛。
Indication: Acute stomachache.
〔用法〕 毫针针刺。
Application: Apply filiform needle acupuncture.

6.8.2 胃痛二方
6.8.2 Prescription for Stomachache II

〔组成〕 内关、膈俞、胃俞、商丘。
Points: Neiguan (PC 6), Geshu (BL 17), Weishu (BL 21), Shanqiu (SP 5).
〔来源〕 《针灸逢源》。
Source: Zhenjiu Fen Yuan (The Origin of Acupuncture and Moxibustion).

〔功效〕 活血通络止痛。
Action: Activating blood circulation, dredging the collaterals and relieving pain.

〔主治〕 血瘀型胃痛。
Indication: Stomachache due to blood stagnation.

〔用法〕 针灸均可。
Application: Apply acupuncture or moxibustion.

6.8.3 胃痛三方
6.8.3 Prescription for Stomachache Ⅲ

〔组成〕 神道。
Point: Shendao (DU 11).

〔来源〕 熊源清经验方。
Source: Xong Yuanqin's experience.

〔功效〕 理气止痛。
Action: Regulating the function of Stomach Qi and relieving pain.

〔主治〕 胃脘痛。
Indication: Stomachache.

〔用法〕 指压法。
Application: Apply point-pressing therapy.

6.8.4 胃痛四方
6.8.4 Prescription for Stomachache Ⅳ

〔组成〕 耳穴胃、交感。
Points: Auricular Acupuncture; Points of Stomach and Sympathetic Nerve.

〔来源〕 刘士佩经验方。

Source: Experience of Liu Shipe.

〔功效〕 解痉止痛。

Action: Releasing spasm and relieving pain.

〔主治〕 胃脘痛。

Indication: Stomachache.

〔用法〕 用王不留行籽粘贴压或埋耳针。

Application: Apply point-pressing or embed intradermal needles.

6.9 中暑类方
6.9 Prescriptions for Sunstroke

6.9.1 中暑一方
6.9.1 Prescription for Sunstroke I

〔组成〕 曲池、委中、舌底静脉。

Points: Quchi(LI 11), Weizhong(BL 40), Sublingual vein.

〔来源〕 《潜斋简效方》。

Source: Qianzhai Jian Xiao Fan (Simple and Effective Prescriptions in the Secret Room).

〔功效〕 泄热去毒血。

Action: Eliminating the summer-heat and toxic material.

〔主治〕 中暑昏迷。

Indication: Coma due to sun-stroke.

〔用法〕 三棱针刺络。

Application: Apply pricking puncture with three-edged needle.

6.9.2 中暑二方
6.9.2 Prescription for Sunstroke II

〔组成〕 中冲。
Point:Zhongchong (PC 9).
〔来源〕 司徒铃经验方。
Source:Experience of Prof. Situ Ling.
〔功效〕 清泄暑热,开窍醒神。
Action:Clearing off the summer heat and waking up the patient from the unconsciousness.
〔主治〕 中暑。
Indication:Sun-stroke.
〔用法〕 三棱针刺络放出。
Application:Apply blood-letting with three-edged needle.

6.9.3 中暑三方
6.9.3 Prescription for Sunstroke III

〔组成〕 人中、合谷、内庭、百会、中极、气海。
Points:Renzhong(RN 23),Hegu(LI 4),Neiting(ST 24),Baihui(DU 20),Zhongji(RN 3),Qihai(RN 6).
〔来源〕 《针灸大成》。
Source:Zhenjiu Da Cheng (The Achievements of Acupuncture and Moxibustion).
〔功效〕 开窍回阳救脱。
Action:Waking up patient from unconsciousness, recuperating the depleted Yang Qi.
〔主治〕 暑厥。

Indication: Syncope due to sunstroke.

〔用法〕 针灸并用。

Application: Apply the acupuncture and moxibustion.

6.10 泄泻类方
6.10 Prescriptions for Diarrhea

6.10.1 泄泻一方
6.10.1 Prescription for Diarrhea I

〔组成〕 神阙。

Point: Shenjue(RN 8).

〔来源〕 《扁鹊神应针灸玉龙经》。

Source: Bianque Shenyin Zhenjiu Yu Long Jing (Miracullous Acupuncture and Moxibustion Classic of Jade Dragon of Bianque).

〔功效〕 温中健脾止泄。

Action: Warming the middle burner and invigorating the spleen to stop the diarrhea.

〔主治〕 急慢性泄泻。

Indicat: Chronic or acute diarrhea.

〔用法〕 隔盐灸。

Application: Apply the salt-partition moxibustion.

6.10.2 泄泻二方
6.10.2 Prescription for Diarrhea II

〔组成〕 四缝。

Point: Sifeng (EX-UE 8).

〔来源〕 任义经验方。

Source: Experience of Ren Yi.

〔功效〕 理脾止泻。

Action: Regulating the function of spleen to stop the diarrhea.

〔主治〕 小儿腹泻。

Indication: Infantile diarrhea.

〔用法〕 毫针轻刺、点刺。

Application: Apply slight puncture or spot pricking with a short filiform needle.

6.10.3 泄泻三方
6.10.3 Prescription for Diarrhea Ⅲ

〔组成〕 眼针大肠区、小肠区。

Points: Eye Acupuncture; Large Intestine and Small intestine areas.

〔来源〕 作者验方。

Source: Experience of authors.

〔功效〕 疏调肠腑。

Action: Regulating the function of intestines.

〔主治〕 急性肠炎。

Indication: Acute enteritis.

〔用法〕 毫针横刺。

Application: Apply transverse insertion with a filiform needle.

6.10.4 泄泻四方
6.10.4 Prescription for Diarrhea Ⅳ

〔组成〕 申脉。

Point:Shenmai(BL 62).

〔来源〕 张登部验方。

Source:Experience of Zhang Denbu.

〔功效〕 调和肠胃。

Action:Regulating the function of stomach and intestines.

〔主治〕 急性寒湿泄泻。

Indication:Acute diarrhea differentiated as the cold-dampness.

〔用法〕 艾灸。

Application:Apply moxibustion.

6.10.5 泄泻五方
6.10.5 Prescription for Diarrhea V

〔组成〕 然谷。

Point:Rangu(KI 2).

〔来源〕 《内经》。

Source:Neijing.

〔功效〕 清利湿热。

Action:Eliminating the dampness heat.

〔主治〕 腹胀泄泻。

Indication:Diarrhea and distention in abdomen.

〔用法〕 然谷泻之并出血。

Application:Apply reducing method, then blood-letting.

6.11 便秘类方
6.11 Prescriptions for Constipation

6.11.1 便秘一方
6.11.1 Prescription for Constipation I

〔组成〕 左腹结穴。
Point: Left Fujie(SP 14).
〔来源〕 彭静山验方。
Source: Peng Jingshan's experience.
〔功效〕 通便。
Action: Promoting the movement of bowel.
〔主治〕 便秘。
Indication: Constipation.
〔用法〕 埋皮内针。
Application: Embed the intradermal needle.

6.11.2 便秘二方
6.11.2 Prescription for Constipation II

〔组成〕 照海、支沟。
Point: Zhaohai(KI 6), Zigou(SJ 6).
〔来源〕 《玉龙歌》。
Source: Yu Long Ge (The Songs of Jade Dragon).
〔功效〕 滋阴润肠通便。
Action: Nourishing Yin to lubricate the intestine and promoting the

movement of bowel.

〔主治〕 阴虚便秘。

Indication: Constipation due to Yin insufficiency.

〔用法〕 补照海,泻支沟。

Application: Apply reinforcing method in KI 6 and reducing in SJ 6.

6.11.3 便秘三方
6.11.3 Prescription for Constipation III

〔组成〕 长强、大敦、阳陵泉。

Points: Changqiang (DU 1), Dadun (LR 1), Yanglingquan (GB 34).

〔来源〕《杂病穴法歌》。

Source: Za Bin Xue Fa Ge (Songs of Point Selection for the Treatment of the Internal Diseases).

〔功效〕 清热顺气导滞。

Action: Eliminating heat-evil, activating the Qi circulation and promoting the movement of bowel.

〔主治〕 热秘气秘。

Indication: Constipation due to heat accumualtion or stagnation of Qi.

〔用法〕 毫针泻法。

Application: Apply reducing method with filiform needle.

6.11.4 便秘四方
6.11.4 Prescrition for Constipation IV

〔组成〕 迎香。

Point: Yinxiang(LI 20)

〔来源〕 作者验方。

Source: Experience of Authors.

〔功效〕 通调肠腑。

Action: Regulating the function of intestines

〔主治〕 便秘。

Indication: Constipation.

〔用法〕 毫针针泻或指压。

Applicaction: Apply reducing with the filiform needle or point-pressing with finger.

6.11.5 便秘五方

6.11.5 Prescription for Constipation Ⅴ

〔组成〕 地仓。

Points: Dicang(ST 4).

〔来源〕《外台秘要》。

Source: Wai Tai Mi Yiao (The Medical Secrets of An Official).

〔功效〕 顺气通便。

Action: Promoting the movement of bowel.

〔主治〕 小儿大便不通。

Indication: Constipation of children.

〔用法〕 毫针泻法。

Application: Apply reducing with the filiform needle.

6.12 心悸类方
6.12 Prescriptions for palpitation

6.12.1 心悸一方
6.12.1 Prescription for Palpitation I

〔组成〕 心俞、膏肓俞、足三里。
Points: Xinshu(BL 15), Gaohuangshu(BL 42), Zusanli(ST 36).
〔来源〕 司徒铃教授验方。
Source: Experience of Prof. Situ Ling.
〔功效〕 补益心气。
Action: Replenish Heart Qi.
〔主治〕 心气虚型心悸。
Indication: Palpitation due to Heart Qi deficiency.
〔用法〕 艾灸。
Application: Apply moxibustion.

6.12.2 心悸二方
6.12.2 Prescription for Palpitation II

〔组成〕 眼针心区。
Point: Eye Acupuncture: Heart area.
〔来源〕 彭静山教授验方。
Source: Experience of Prof. Peng Jingshan.
〔功效〕 宁心安神。
Action: Tranquilizing.

〔主治〕 各种原因引起心悸。

Indication: Palpitation due to a varety of causes.

〔用法〕 毫针针刺。

Application: Apply puncture of filiform needle.

6.12.3 心悸三方
6.12.3 Prescription for Palpitation Ⅲ

〔组成〕 胆俞、解溪。

Points: Danshu(BL 19), Jiexi(ST 41).

〔来源〕 《神灸经纶》。

Source: Shenjiu Jinglun(Treatise of Miracullous Moxibustion).

〔功效〕 清热化痰,和胃降浊。

Action: Eliminating the heat and phlegm, lowering the adversely rising turbid fluid.

〔主治〕 痰热内蕴引起心悸。

Indication: Palpitation due to accumulation of heat and phlegm.

〔用法〕 毫针泻法。

Application: Apply reducing method with filiform needle.

6.13 心痛类方
6.13 Prescriptions for precordial pain

6.13.1 心痛一方
6.13.1 Prescription for Precordial Pain Ⅰ

〔组成〕 支沟、太溪、然谷。

Points: Zigou(SJ 6), Taixi(KI 3), Rangu(KI 2).

〔来源〕《千金方》。

Source: Valuble Prescriptions(Qian Jin Yiao Fan).

〔功效〕 祛寒活血通阳。

Action: Dispelling cold and activating circulation of blood and Yang Qi.

〔主治〕 心痛如锥刺。

Indication: Precordial pain.

〔用法〕 针灸并用。

Application: Apply both acupuncture and moxibustion.

6.13.2 心痛二方

6.13.2 Prescription for Precordial Pain II

〔组成〕 涌泉、太冲。

Points: Yongquan(KI 1), Taichong(LR 3).

〔来源〕《针灸逢源》

Source: Zhenjiu Feng Yuan (The Origin of Acupuncture and Moxistion).

〔功效〕 理气止痛。

Action: Activating circulaion of Qi and relieving pain.

〔主治〕 心痛。

Indication: Precordial pain.

〔用法〕 毫针泻法。

Application: Apply reducing method with filiform needle.

6.13.3 心痛三方
6.13.3 Prescription for Precordial Pain Ⅲ

〔组成〕 内关、膻中、然谷。
Points: Neiguan(PC 6), Tangzhong(RN 17), Rangu(KI 2).

〔来源〕 贺普仁经验方。
Source: Experience of He Puren.

〔功效〕 调补心阳,理气活血止痛。
Action: Tonifying the Yang energy of Heart, activating circulanton of blood and Qi, and relieving pain.

〔主治〕 心阳不振、气滞血瘀引起心痛。
Indication: Precordial pain due to deficiency of Heart Yang or due to stagnation of blood and Qi.

〔用法〕 针内关、膻中,然谷刺络。
Application: Apply acupuncture in Neiguan (PC 6), and Tangzhong (RN 17); apply spot pricking puncture in Rangu(KI 2).

6.13.4 心痛四方
6.13.4 Prescription for Precordial Pain Ⅳ

〔组成〕 印堂、心俞、至阳。
Points: Yintang(EX-HN 3), Xinshu(BL 15), Zhiyang(DU 9).

〔来源〕 作者验方。
Source: Authors' experience.

〔功效〕 活血通脉止痛。
Action: Activating circulation of blood and dredging the collaterals, relieving pain.

〔主治〕 心绞痛。

Indication: Angina pectoris.

〔用法〕 针刺至阳、印堂,艾灸心俞。

Application: Apply acupuncture in EX-HN 3 and DU 9, moxibustion in Xinshu(BL 15).

6.13.5 心痛五方
6.13.5 Prescription for Precordial Pain V

〔组成〕 内关、足三里、膻中。

Points: Neiguan(PC 6), Zusanli(ST 36), Tangzhong(RN 17).

〔来源〕 朱柏君《中国针灸》1986(5)。

Source: Zu Baijun 1986(5) Chinese Acupuncture and Moxibustion.

〔功效〕 益气活血。

Action: Tonifying Qi and activating blood circulation.

〔主治〕 冠心病、心绞痛。

Indication: Angina pectoris and coronary heart disease.

〔用法〕 艾灸。

Application: Moxibustion.

6.14 胁痛类方
6.14 Prescriptions for Hypochondriac Pain

6.14.1 胁痛一方
6.14.1 Prescription for Hypochondriac Pain I

〔组成〕 阳陵泉、阿是。

Points: Yanglingquan(GB 34), Ashi points.

〔来源〕 作者验方。

Source: Experience of authors.

〔功效〕 清利肝胆湿热。

Action: Eliminating the dampness heat in liver and gallbladder.

〔主治〕 肋间神经痛。

Indication: Intercostal neuralgia.

〔用法〕 针泻阳陵泉,肋部痛点埋皮内针。

Application: Apply reducing in GB 34 and embed intradermal needle in Ashi points.

6.14.2 胁痛二方
6.14.2 Prescription for Hypochondriac Pain Ⅱ

〔组成〕 行间、足三里。

Points: Xingjian(LR 2), Zusanli(ST 36).

〔来源〕 《内经》。

Source: Neijing.

〔功效〕 疏肝理气和胃。

Action: Disperssing stagnated liver energy and regulating the function of stomach.

〔主治〕 两胁痛。

Indication: Bilateral hypochondriac pain.

〔用法〕 泻行间、补足三里。

Application: Apply reducing method in LR 2 and reinforcing method in ST 36.

6.14.3 胁痛三方
6.14.3 Prescription for Hgpochondriac Pain Ⅲ

〔组成〕 足窍阴。
Points: Zuqiaoyin(GB 44).
〔来源〕 《全生指迷方》。
Source: Quan Sheng Zhi Mi Fang (Guiding Prescriptions).
〔功效〕 祛瘀通络。
Action: Removing blood stasis and dredging the collaterals.
〔主治〕 胁痛不得息
Indication: Hypochondriac pain with diffculty to breathe.
〔用法〕 毫针泻法。
Application: Apply reducing method with filiform needle.

6.14.4 胁痛四方
6.14.4 Prescription for Hypochondriac Pain Ⅳ

〔组成〕 太冲、足三里。
Points: Taichong(LR 3), Zusanli(ST 36).
〔来源〕 作者验方。
Source: Experience of Authors.
〔功效〕 疏肝理气,健脾胃。
Action: Dispelling stagnated liver energy and invigorating the spleen.
〔主治〕 肝炎引起胁痛。
Indication: Hypochondriac pain caused by heratitis.
〔用法〕 泻太冲,补足三里
Application: Apply reducing in LR 3 and reinforcing in ST 36.

6.15 失眠类方
6.15 Prescription for Insomnia.

6.15.1 失眠一方
6.15.1 Prescription for Insomnia Ⅰ

〔组成〕 申脉、照海、印堂。
Points: Shenmai(BL 62), Zhaohai(KI 6), Yintang(EX-HN 3).
〔来源〕 作者验方。
Source: Experience of authors.
〔功效〕 调整阴阳,镇静安神。
Action: Tranquilizing to reach the equilibrium between Yin and Yang.
〔主治〕 失眠。
Indication: Insomnia.
〔用法〕 泻申脉,补照海,泻印堂。
Application: Apply reducing method in Shenmai(BL 62) and Yintang (EX-HN 3) and reinforcing in Zhaohai(KI 6).

6.15.2 失眠二方
6.15.2 Prescription for Insomnia Ⅱ

〔组成〕 阴交、谚禧。
Points: Yinjiao(RN 7), Yixi(BL 45).
〔来源〕 《针灸集成》。
Source: Zhenjiu Ji Cheng (A Collection of Acupuncture and Moxi-

bustion Works).

〔功效〕 导阳入阴,安神。
Action：Inducing Yang into Yin and tranquilizing.
〔主治〕 失眠。
Indication：Insomnia.
〔用法〕 艾灸。
Application：Moxibustion.

6.15.3 失眠三方
6.15.3 Prescription for Insomnia Ⅳ

〔组成〕 涌泉。
Points：Yongquan(KI 1).
〔来源〕 查少农验方。
Source：Cha Shaonong's experience.
〔功效〕 补肾宁神。
Action：Reinforcing the kidney and tranquilizing.
〔主治〕 失眠、心悸。
Indication：Insomnia and palpitation.
〔用法〕 艾灸。
Application：Moxibustion.

6.15.4 失眠 4 方
6.15.4 Prescription for Insomnia Ⅳ

〔组成〕 心俞、肾俞、神门、三阴交。
Points：Xinshu(BL 15), Shenshu(BL 23), shenmen(HT 7), Sanyinjiao(SP 6).
〔来源〕 《陆瘦燕针灸医著医案选》。

Source: Lu Shouyan Zhenjiu Yi Ji Xiang (The Cases Selection Treated with Acupuncture and Moxibustion by Lushouyan).

〔功效〕 交通心肾。
Action: Harmonizing the heart and the kidney.

〔主治〕 心肾不交引起失眠
Indication: Insomnia due to disharmony between the kidney and heart.

〔用法〕 心俞用灸,肾俞、三阴交用补法,神门泻法。
Application: Apply moxibustion in Xinshu, reinforcing method in Sanyinjiao and Shenshu; and reducing method in Shenmen with acupuncture.

6.16 高血压眩晕类方
6.16 Prescriptions for Dizziness due to Hypertension

6.16.1 高血压一方
6.16.1 Prescription for Dizziness due to Hypertension I

〔组成〕 膈俞。
Point: Geshu (BL 17).

〔来源〕 彭静山教授验方。
Source: Prof. Peng Jingshan's experience.

〔功效〕 活血降压。
Action: Activating blood circulation and lowering the blood pressure

〔主治〕 高血压。

Indication: Hypertension.

〔用法〕 埋皮针。

Application: Embed intradermal needle.

6.16.2 高血压二方
6.16.2 Prescription for Dizziness due to Hypertension II

〔组成〕 四关穴。

Points: Four-gates points (Bilateral LI 4 and LR 3).

〔来源〕 作者验方。

Source: Experience of authors.

〔功效〕 平肝熄风

Action: Calming the liver to inhibit the endogenous wind.

〔主治〕 高血压眩晕。

Indication: Dizziness due to hypertension.

〔用法〕 毫针泻法。

Application: Apply reducing method with filiform needle.

6.16.3 高血压三方
6.16.3 Prescription for Dizziness due to Hypertension III

〔组成〕 百会。

Point: Baihui (DU 20).

〔来源〕 司徒铃教授验方。

Source: Experience of Prof. Situ Ling.

〔功效〕 祛痰降浊平肝。

Action: Eliminating phlegm, lowering adverse rising turbid fluid and calming liver.

〔主治〕 高血压眩晕(痰浊型)。

Indication: Dizziness due to hypertension, differentiated as phlegm and turbid fluid accumulation.

〔用法〕 压灸。

Application: Apply moxibustion, direct moxibustion with a moxa cone, then pressing and extinguishing with a moxa stick to let the warm sensation penetrate downwards.

6.16.4 高血压四方
6.16.4 Preseription for Dizziness due to Hypertension Ⅳ

〔组成〕 印堂,素髎。
Points: Yintang(EX-HN 3), Suliao(DU 25).

〔来源〕 彭静山教授验方。
Source: Experience of Prof. Peng Jingshan.

〔功效〕 调降血压。
Action: Lowering the blood Pressure.

〔主治〕 高血压。
Indication: Hypertension.

〔用法〕 毫针泻法。
Application: Apply reducing method with filiform needle.

6.16.5 高血压五方
6.16.5 Prescription for Dizziness due to Hypertension Ⅴ

〔组成〕 肩井、丰隆。
Point: Jianjing(GB 21), Fenglong(ST 40).

〔来源〕 作者验方。
Source: Experience of authors.

〔功效〕 祛痰降浊,利胆降压。

Action: Eliminating phlegm and lowering the adversely rising turbid fluid, regulating function of gallbladder, and lowering the blood pressure.

〔主治〕 高血压。

Indication: Hypertension.

〔用法〕 毫针泻法。

Application: Apply reducing method with filiform needle.

6.17 头痛类方
6.17 Prescriptions for Headache

6.17.1 头痛一方
6.17.1 Prescription for Headache I

〔组成〕 强间、丰隆。

Points: Qiangjian (DU 18), Fenglong (ST 40).

〔来源〕 《百证赋》。

Source: Baizhenfu (The Poems About the Acupuncture Treatment of Syndromes).

〔功效〕 涤痰镇痛。

Action: Eliminating phlegm to relieve pain.

〔主治〕 痰浊头痛。

Indication: Headache differentiated as phlegm and turbid fluid.

〔用法〕 毫针泻法。

Application: Apply reducing method with filiform needle.

6.17.2 头痛二方
6.17.2 Prescription for Headache II

〔组成〕 四花穴、医风。
Points: Four flowers points (Bilatetal BL 17 and BL 19), Yifeng (SJ 17).

〔来源〕 司徒铃教授验方。
Source: Experience of Situ Ling.

〔功效〕 活血化瘀,疏调少阳。
Action: Activating circulation of blood and Qi, and regulating the Shaoyang meridian.

〔主治〕 偏头痛。
Indication: Migraine.

〔用法〕 挑治。
Application: Apply pricking therapy.

6.17.3 头痛三方
6.17.3 Prescription for Headache III

〔组成〕 四关穴、百会。
Points: Four-gate\points (Bilateral LI 4 and LR 3), Baihui (DU 20).

〔来源〕 作者验方。
Source: Experience of authors.

〔功效〕 平肝潜阳,祛风止痛。
Action: Calming the liver, dispelling the wind and relieving pain.

〔主治〕 巅顶头胀痛。
Indication: Distending pain at the vertex of the head.

〔用法〕 四关用毫针泻法,百会用三棱针刺络。

Application: Apply reducing method in four-gate points and spot pricking puncture in Baihui(DU 20).

6.17.4 头痛四方
6.17.4 Prescripton for Headache Ⅳ

〔组成〕 太阳、足临泣,中渚。

Points: Taiyang(EX-HN 5), Zulingqi(GB 41), Zhongzhu(SJ 3).

〔来源〕 作者验方。

Source: Experience of authors.

〔功效〕 祛风活血通络。

Action: Expelling the wind, activating blood circulation and dredging the collaterals.

〔主治〕 偏头痛。

Indication: Migraine.

〔用法〕 太阳刺络,足临泣、中渚均用毫针泻之。

Application: Apply spot pricking therapy in Taiyang(EX-HN 5) and reducing method in other points.

6.17.5 头痛五方
6.17.5 Prescription for Headache Ⅴ

〔组成〕 痛点缪刺。

Point: Ashi Point.

〔来源〕 彭静山教授验方。

Source: Experience of Peng Jingshan.

〔功效〕 通络止痛。

Action: Dredging the collaterals and relieving pain.

〔主治〕 偏头痛。

Indication: Migraine.

〔用法〕 先找最痛点,再在健侧对应点刺。

Appncation: Find the most painful point in affected side of head, the apply spot pricking at its symmetric point in heathly side.

6.17.6 头痛六方
6.17.6 Prescription for Headache Ⅵ

〔组成〕 风池、合谷、丝竹空。

Points: Fengchi(GB 20), Hegu(LI 4), Sizukong(SJ 23).

〔来源〕 《针灸大成》。

Source: Zhenjiu Da Cheng (The Achievements of Acupuncture and Moxibustion).

〔功效〕 祛风止痛。

Action: Expelling the wind and relieving pain.

〔主治〕 偏头痛。

Indication: Migraine.

〔用法〕 毫针泻法。

Application: Apply reducing method with filiform needle.

6.18 癫痫类方
6.18 Prescriptions for Epilepsy

6.18.1 癫痫一方
6.18.1 Prescription for Epilepsy Ⅰ

〔组成〕 天柱。
Point: Tianzhu(BL 10).
〔来源〕 《内经》。
Source: Neijing.
〔功效〕 豁痰熄风醒神。
Action: Eliminating the phlegm and calming endogenous wind, and waking up the patient from unconsciousness.
〔主治〕 癫痫发作。
Indication: Attack of epilepsy.
〔用法〕 毫针泻之。
Application: Apply reducing method with the filiform needle.

6.18.2 癫痫二方
6.18.2 Prescription for Epilepsy Ⅱ

〔组成〕 鸠尾、中脘、列缺、照海。
Points: Jiuwei(RN 15), Zhongwan(RN 12), Lieque(Lu 7), Zhaohai(KI 6).
〔来源〕 作者验方。
Source: Experience of authors.

〔功效〕 健脾化痰定痫。
Action: Invigorating the spleen and eliminating phlegm, controlling the attack of epilepsy.

〔主治〕 癫痫夜晚发作者。
Indication: Noctural attack of epilepsy.

〔用法〕 鸠尾透中脘,列缺用泻法,照海用补法。
Application: Apply penetrating puncture technique from point RN 15 to RN 12 with reducing method; reducing method in Lieque(LU 7) and reinforcing method in Zhaohai(KI 6).

6.18.3 癫痫三方
6.18.3 Prescription for Epilepsy III

〔组成〕 人中、阴交、申脉、照海。
Points: Renzhong(DU 26), Yinjiao(RN 7), shenmai(BL 62), Zhaohai(KI 6).

〔来源〕 《脾胃论》。
Source: Piwei Lun (Treaties on the Spleen and Stomach).

〔功效〕 调奇经开窍定痫。
Action: Regulating the extraordinary meridians, waking up patient from unconciousness, and controlling the attack of epilepsy.

〔主治〕 癫痫。
Indication: Epilepsy.

〔用法〕 毫针泻之。
Application: Apply reducing method with filiform needle.

6.18.4 癫痫四方
6.18.4 Prescription for Epilepsy IV

〔组成〕 四关、内关。
Points: Four-gate points (Bilateral LI4 and LR3), Neiguan (PC 6).

〔来源〕 作者验方。
Source: Experience of authors.

〔功效〕 熄风定痫止痛。
Action: Calming endogenous wind, controlling the epilepitic attack, relieving pain.

〔主治〕 癫痫头痛。
Indication: Epileptic headache.

〔用法〕 毫针泻之。
Application: Apply reducing method with filiform needle.

6.18.5 癫痫五方
6.18.5 Prescription for Epilepsy V

〔组成〕 长强、腰奇、鸠尾。
Points: Changqiang (DU 1), Yaoqi (Ex-B 9), Jiuqei (RN 15).

〔来源〕 司徒铃验方。
Source: Experience of Situ Ling.

〔功效〕 豁痰熄风定痫。
Action: Eliminating phlegm, calming endogenous wind, and controlling the attack of epilepsy.

〔主治〕 癫痫。
Indication: Epilepsy.

〔用法〕 毫针泻法。

Application: Apply reducing method with filiform needle.

6.19 消渴类方
6.19 Prescriptions for Diabetes

6.19.1 消渴一方
6.19.1 Prescription for Diabetes I

〔组成〕 承浆、意舍、关冲、然谷。

Points: Chenjiang(RN 24), Yishe(BL 49), Guangchong(SJ 1), Rangu(KI 2).

〔来源〕《普济方》

Source: Puji Fang (Experiential Prescriptions for Curing All People).

〔功效〕 清热润燥生津。

Action: Clearing off heat, moisturizing the dryness and promoting the production of body fluid.

〔主治〕 消渴

Indication: Diabetes.

〔用法〕 毫针泻法。

Application: Apply reducing method with filiform needle.

6.19.2 消渴二方
6.19.2 Prescription for Diabetes II

〔组成〕 涌泉、太溪。

Points: Rongquan(KI 1), Taixi(KI 3).

〔来源〕 徐笨人验方。

Source: Experience of Xu Banren.

〔功效〕 养阴益肾。

Action: Nourishing the Yin and benefiting the kidney.

〔主治〕 糖尿病。

Indication: Diabetes.

〔用法〕 磁锤叩打,每穴 50 次左右。

Application: Apply hammering with magnetic hammer for about 50 times at each points.

6.19.3 消渴三方
6.19.3 Prescription for Diabetes Ⅲ

〔组成〕 鱼际、内庭、太溪、关元、胰俞。

Points: Yuji(LU 10), Neiting(ST 44), Taixi(KI 3), Guanyuan (RN 4), Yishu point(Back-shu point of pancreas, at the level of 8th thoracic vertebra, beside the middle line of back).

〔来源〕 作者验方。

Source: Experience of authors.

〔功效〕 清热养阴补肾。

Action: Clearing off the heat and nourishing the Yin and reinforcing the kidney.

〔主治〕 糖尿病。

Indication: Diabetes.

〔用法〕 鱼际、内庭用泻法,太溪、关元用补法,胰俞埋针。

Application: Apply reducing method in Yuji(LU 10) and Neiting (ST 44), reinforcing method in Taixi(KI 3), Guanyuang(RN 4);

then embed the intradermal needle in Yishu.

6.20 肩周炎类方
6.20 Prescriptions for Periarthritis of Shoulder

6.20.1 肩痛一方
6.20.1 Prescription for Periarithritis of Shoulder I

〔组成〕 阳陵泉、太冲
Points: Yanglingquan(GB 34), Taichong(LR 3).
〔来源〕 吕景山经验方。
Source: Experience of Ru Jingshan.
〔功效〕 理气活血舒筋。
Action: Activating the circulation of Qi and blood, and relaxing tendons.
〔主治〕 肩周炎。
Indication: Periarthritis of shoulder.
〔用法〕 毫针泻法。
Application: Apply the reducing method with filiform needle.

6.20.2 肩痛二方
6.20.2 Prescription for Periarthritis of Shoulder II

〔组成〕 天鼎、天柱。
Points: Tianding(LI 1), Tianzhu(BL 10).
〔来源〕 方幼安验方。
Source: Experience of Fang Youan.

〔功效〕 通络止痛。

Action: Dredging the collaterals and relieving pain.

〔主治〕 肩痛。

Indication: Pain of shoulder joint.

〔用法〕 毫针泻法。

Application: Apply reducing method with filiform needle.

6.20.3 肩痛三方
6.20.3 Prescription for Periarthritis of Shouder III

〔组成〕 养老、天柱。

Points: Yanglao(SI 6), Tainzhu(BL 10).

〔来源〕 《千金方》。

Source: Qian Jin Fang (Valuable Prescriptions).

〔功效〕 祛湿通络。

Action: Eliminating the dampness and dredging the collaterals.

〔主治〕 肩痛如折。

Indication: Pain in shoulder joint as if that in fracture.

〔用法〕 毫针泻之。

Application: Apply reducing method with filiform needle.

6.20.4 肩痛四方
6.20.4 Prescription for Periarthritis of Shoulder IV

〔组成〕 眼上焦、条口透承山。

Points: Eye Acupuncture: Upper burner area, Tiaokou(ST 38), Changshan(BL 65).

〔来源〕 作者验方。

Source: Experience of authors.

〔功效〕 疏调气血,舒筋利肩。

Action: Regulating the circulation of blood and Qi, relaxing the tendons and benefiting the shoulder joint.

〔主治〕 肩痛。

Indication: Pain in shoulder joint.

〔用法〕 先针眼上焦,后针体穴均泻法。

Application: Needle eye acupoint at first, then apply penetrating puncture technique from Tiaokou(ST 38) to Chengshan(BL 65) with reducing method.

6.20.5 肩痛五方

6.20.5 Prescription for Periarthritis of Shoulder V

〔组成〕 肩三针、大椎、膈俞。

Points: Jianyu(LI 5), Jianquan(1 cun above the end of anterior axillary wrinkle), Jianhou(1.5cun above the end of posterior axillary wrinkle) Dazhui(DU 14), Geshu(BL 17).

〔来源〕 作者验方。

Source: Experience of authors.

〔功效〕 散寒祛湿,活血止痛。

Action: Dispelling the cold and dampness, activating the circulation of blood and relieving pain.

〔主治〕 寒湿型肩周炎。

Indication: Periarthritis differentiated as type cold-dampness.

〔用法〕 火针点刺。

Application: Apply spot prickling with burning needle.

6.21 落枕类方
6.21 Prescriptions for Torticollis

6.21.1 落枕一方
6.21.1 Prescription for Torticollis Ⅰ

〔组成〕 列缺、后溪。
Points: Lieque(LU 7), Houxi(SI 3).
〔来源〕 司徒铃验方。
Sorrce: Experience of Situ Ling.
〔功效〕 祛寒湿,活血舒筋。
Action: Dispelling the cold and dampeness, activating the circulation of blood and relaxing tendons.
〔主治〕 落枕。
Indication: Torticollis.
〔用法〕 毫针泻法。
Application: Apply reducing method with filiform needle.

6.21.2 落枕2方
6.21.2 Prscription for Torticollis Ⅱ

〔组成〕 后溪、束骨。
Points: Houxi(SI 3), Shugu(BL 65).
〔来源〕 《内经》。
Source: Neijing.
〔功效〕 舒筋活络。

Action: Relaxing the tendons and dredging the collaterals.

〔主治〕 落枕项痛不可以顾,不可俯仰。

Indication: Pain and impaired movement of the neck due to torticollis.

〔用法〕 毫针泻法。

Application: Apply ruducing method with filiform needle.

6.21.3 落枕三方
6.21.3 Prescription for Torticollis Ⅲ

〔组成〕 后溪、合谷、承浆。

Points: Houxi(SI 3), Hegu(LI 4), Chengjiang(RN 24).

〔来源〕 《针灸大成》。

Source: Zhenjiu Da Cheng (The Achievements of Acupuncture and Moxibustion).

〔功效〕 祛风通络。

Action: Dispelling wind and dredging the collaterals.

〔主治〕 颈项难转。

Indication: Impaired movement of the neck due to torticollis.

〔用法〕 毫针泻法。

Application: Apply reducing method with filiform needle.

5.21.4 落枕四方
6.21.4 Prescription for Taticouis Ⅳ

〔组成〕 承浆、风府。

Points: Chengjiang(RN 24), Fengfu(DU 26).

〔来源〕 《针方六集》。

Source: Zhen Fang Liu Ji (The Six Chapters of Acupuncture Prescriptions).

〔功效〕 祛风通络。
Action: Dispelling the wind and dredging the collaterals.

〔主治〕 颈项强痛,回顾难。
Indication: Stiffness, pain and impaired movement of neck.

〔用法〕 毫针泻法。
Application: Apply reducing method with filiform needle.

6.21.5 落枕五方
6.21.5 Prescription for Torticollis V

〔组成〕 中渚。
Point: Zhongzhu(SJ 3).

〔来源〕 戴铁城验方。
Soource: Experience of Dai Tiecheng.

〔功效〕 舒筋止痛。
Action: Relaxing the tendons and relieving the pain.

〔主治〕 落枕。
Indication: Torticollis.

〔用法〕 毫针泻法。
Application: Apply reducing method with filiform needle.

6.21.6 落枕六方
6.21.6 Prescription for Torticollis VI

〔组成〕 阳陵泉。
Point: Yanglingquan(GB 34).

〔来源〕 赵福成《贵阳中医学院学报》1987(2)。
Source: Zhao Fucheng 1987(2) Journal of Guiyang TCM Col-

lege.

〔功效〕 舒筋通络。
Action: Relaxing tendons and dredging the collaterals.
〔主治〕 落枕。
Indication: Torticollis.
〔用法〕 毫针泻法。
Application: Apply reducing method with filiform needle.

6.21.7 落枕七方
6.21.7 Prescription for Torticollis Ⅶ

〔组成〕 耳穴颈、神门。
Points: Auricular point: Neck and Shenmen.
〔来源〕 夏金陵《中医杂志》1985(5)。
Source: Xia Jinling 1985(5) Journal of TCM.
〔功效〕 通络止痛。
Action: Dredging the collaterals and relieving pain.
〔主治〕 落枕。
Indication: Torticollis.
〔用法〕 用绿豆放在伤湿止痛膏上贴于耳穴按压。
Application: Apply point-pressing in auricular points.

6.21.8 落枕八方
6.21.8 Prescription for Torticolis Ⅷ

〔组成〕 眼针上焦。
Point: Eye acupuncture: upper burner area.
〔来源〕 彭静山验方。
Source: Experience of Peng Jingshan.

〔功效〕 祛风止痛。
Action: Dispelling the wind and relieving pain.

〔主治〕 落枕。
Indication: Torticollis.

〔用法〕 毫针针刺。
Application: Apply the acupuncture with filiform needle.

6.21.9 落枕九方
6.21.9 Prescription for Torticollis Ⅸ

〔组成〕 落枕穴(手背食指掌指关节尺侧缘)。
Point: Torticollis point in Hand-acupuncture(On the back of hand, at the ulnar side of metacarpophalangeal joint of index finger).

〔来源〕《手针新疗法》。
Source: Shou Zhen Xin Liao Fa (New Therapeutic Technique of Hand Acupuncture.)

〔功效〕 止痛。
Action: Relieving pain.

〔主治〕 落枕。
Indication: Torticollis.

〔用法〕 毫针泻法。
Application: Apply reducing method with filiform needle.

6.21.10 落枕十方
6.21.10 Prescription for Torticollis Ⅹ

〔组成〕 内关。
point: Neiguan(PC 6).

〔来源〕 骆汉成《中级医刊》1990(10)

Source: Lou Hancheng 1990(10) Zhongji Yi Kan (Journal of Continual Medical Education).

〔功效〕 活血止痛。

Action: Activating the circulation of the blood and relieving pain.

〔主治〕 落枕。

Indication: Torticollis.

〔用法〕 毫针泻法。

Application: Apply reducing method with filiform needle.

6.21.11 落枕十一方
6.21.11 Prescription for Torticollis XI

〔组成〕 悬钟。

Point: Xuanzhong(GB 39).

〔来源〕 谷端起《中级医刊》1990(10)。

Source: Gu Duanqi 1991(10) Zhongji Yi Kan (Journal of Continual Medical Education).

〔功效〕 祛风调经止痛。

Action: Dispelling the wind and regulating the circulation of meridians and relieving pain.

〔主治〕 落枕。

Indication: Torticollis.

〔用法〕 毫针泻法。

Application: Apply reducing method with filiform needle.

6.22 痛经类方
6.22 Prescriptions for Dysmenorrhea

6.22.1 痛经一方
6.22.1 Prescription for Dysmenorrhea I

〔组成〕 手足中指尖。
Points: The tip of middle finger and middle toe.
〔来源〕 周楣声验方。
Source: Zhou Meisheng's experience.
〔功效〕 活血止痛。
Action: Activating the circulation of blood and relieving pain.
〔主治〕 痛经难忍。
Indication: Dysmenorrhea, intolerable abdominal pain.
〔用法〕 毫针泻法。
Application: Apply reducing method with filiform needle.

6.22.2 痛经二方
6.22.2 Prescription for Dysmenorrhea II

〔组成〕 公孙、关元。
Points: Gongsun (SP 4), Guanyuan (RN 4).
〔来源〕 王品山验方。
Source: Wang Pinshan's experience.
〔功效〕 行气活血,调冲补肾。
Action: Activating circulation of the blood and Qi, regulating the

function of Chong meridian and reinforcing the kidney.

〔主治〕 痛经。
Indication: Dysmenorrhea.
〔用法〕 毫针针刺。
Application: Apply the acupuncture with filiform needle.

6.22.3 痛经三方
6.22.3 Prescription for Dysmenorrhea Ⅲ

〔组成〕 人中、八髎。
Points: Renzhong(DU 26), Baliao(BL 31,32,33,34).
〔来源〕 作者验方。
Sorrce: Experience of authors.
〔功效〕 行气活血,祛寒止痛。
Action: Activating circulation of the blood and Qi, dispelling cold, relieving pain.
〔主治〕 痛经。
Indication: Dysmenorrhea.
〔用法〕 人中泻法,八髎艾灸。
Application: Apply reducing method in Renzhong and moxibustion in Baliao points.

6.22.4 痛经四方
6.22.4 Prescription for Dysmenorrhea Ⅳ

〔组成〕 承山。
point: Chengshan(BL 57).
〔来源〕 田凤鸣、田旭光《河北中医》1985(6)。
Source: Tian Fengming and Tian Xugunag 1985(6) Hebai Jour-

nal of TCM.

〔功效〕 行气活血止痛。
Action: Activating circulation of blood and Qi.

〔主治〕 痛经。
Indication: Dysmenorrhea.

〔用法〕 毫针泻法。
Application: Apply reducing method.

6.22.5 痛经五方
6.22.5 Prescription for Dysmenorrhea V

〔组成〕 气海、三阴交。
Points: Qihai(RN 6), Sanyinjiao(SP 6).

〔来源〕 《针灸逢源》。
Source: Zhenjiu Feng Yuan (The Origin of Acupuncture and Moxibustion).

〔功效〕 调补肝肾,散寒止痛。
Action: Reinforcing the kidney and liver, dispelling the cold and relieving pain.

〔主治〕 痛经。
Indication: Dysmenorrhea.

〔用法〕 针灸并用。
Application: Apply both moxibustion and acupuncture.

6.22.6 痛经六方
6.22.6 Prescription for Dysmenorrhea VI

〔组成〕 四关、关元。
Point: Four-gate points (Bilateral LI4 and LR3) Guanyuan (RN

4).

〔来源〕 作者验方。
Source: Experience of authors.
〔功效〕 理气活血止痛。
Action: Activating circulation of blood and Qi, relieving pain.
〔主治〕 痛经。
Indication: Dysmenorrhea.
〔用法〕 泻四关,艾灸关元。
Application: Apply reducing method in four-gate points and moxibustion in RN 4.

6.22.7 痛经七方
6.22.7 Prescription for Dysmenorrhea Ⅶ

〔组成〕 眼肝区。
Point: Eye acupuncture; Liver area.
〔来源〕 作者验方。
Source: Experience of author.
〔功效〕 理气行血散寒。
Action: Activating circulation of the blood and Qi, dispelling the cold.
〔主治〕 痛经。
Indication: Dysmenorrhea.
〔用法〕 毫针针刺。
Application: Apply acupuncture with filiform needle.

6.23 闭经类方
6.23 Prescriptions for Amenorrhea

6.23.1 闭经一方
6.23.1 Prescription for Amenorrhea I

〔组成〕 腰俞、照海。
Points: Yaoshu(DU 2), Zhaohai(KI 6).

〔来源〕 《神灸经纶》。
Source: Shenjiu Jing Lun (The Treatise of Miracullous Moxibustion).

〔功效〕 补肾行血调经。
Action: Tonifying the kidney, activating the blood circulation and regulating the menstruation.

〔主治〕 闭经。
Indication: Amenorrhea.

〔用法〕 艾灸。
Application: Apply moxibustion.

6.23.2 闭经二方
6.23.2 Prescription for Amenorrhea II

〔组成〕 合谷、阴交、血海、气冲。
Points: Hegu(LI 4), Yinjiao(RN 7), Zhaohai(SP 10), Qichong(ST 30).

〔来源〕 《针灸集成》。

Source: Zhenjiu Ji Cheng (A Collection of Acupuncture and Moxibustion Therapy).

〔功效〕 理气活血行滞。

Action: Activating circulation of the blood and Qi.

〔主治〕 闭经。

Indication: Amenorrhea.

〔用法〕 毫针针刺。

Application: Apply acupuncture with filiform needle.

6.23.3 闭经三方
6.23.3 Prescription for Amenorrhea Ⅲ

〔组成〕 四关、血海、中极。

Points: Four-gate points (bilateral LI 4 and LR 3), Xuehai (SP 10), Zhongji (RN 3).

〔来源〕 作者验方。

Source: Experience of authors.

〔功效〕 活血祛瘀,理气通经。

Action: Activating the circulation of the blood and Qi, removing the blood stasis.

〔主治〕 气滞血瘀型闭经。

Indication: Amenorrhea due to the stagnation of the blood and Qi.

〔用法〕 毫针泻法。

Application: Apply reducing method with filiform needle.

6.24 崩漏类方
6.24 Prescriptions for Uterine Bleeding

6.24.1 崩漏1方
6.24.1 Prescription for Uterine Bleeding Ⅰ

〔组成〕 隐白。
Point: Yinbai(SP 1).
〔来源〕 《金针梅花诗钞》。
Source: Jin Zhen Meihua Shi Cao (The Poems Collection of Golden Acupuncture Needle).
〔功效〕 益气固本,养血止血。
Action: Invigorating Qi and strengthening the essence, invigorating the blood and stopping bleeding.
〔主治〕 崩漏。
Indication: Uterine bleeding.
〔用法〕 艾灸。
Application: Apply moxibustion.

6.24.2 崩漏二方
6.24.2 Prescription for Uterine Bleeding Ⅱ

〔组成〕 通里。
Point: Tongli(HT 5).
〔来源〕 《医宗金鉴》。
Source: Yi Zong Jin Jian (The Gold Mirror of Medicine).

〔功效〕 清热凉血,固经涩血。

Action: Clearing off heat and cooling the blood, stopping the uterine bleeding.

〔主治〕 崩漏。

Indication: Uterine bleeding.

〔用法〕 毫针泻法。

Application: Apply reducing method with filiform needle.

6.24.3 崩漏三方
6.24.3 Prescription for Uterine Bleeding Ⅲ

〔组成〕 气海、中极、照海。

Points: Qihai(RN 6), Zhongji(RN 3), Zhaohai(KI 6).

〔来源〕 《神灸经纶》。

Source: Shenjiu Jing Lun (Classic Protocol of Moxibustion).

〔功效〕 补肾止血。

Action: Invigorating the kidney and stopping bleeding.

〔主治〕 崩漏。

Indication: Uterine bleeding.

〔用法〕 针灸并用。

Application: Apply moxibustion and acupuncture.

6.24.4 崩漏四方
6.24.4 Prescription for Uterine Bleeding Ⅳ

〔组成〕 大敦。

Point: Dadun(LR 1).

〔来源〕 《铜人腧穴针灸图经》。

Source: Tongren Shuxue Zhenjiu Tujing (Illustrated Manual on the Points for Acupuncture and Moxibustion as Found on the Bronze Figure).

〔功效〕 调肝止血。
Action: Regulating function of liver and stopping uterine bleeding.

〔主治〕 妇人血崩不止。
Indication: Persistent uterine bleeding.

〔用法〕 针灸并用。
Applicaton: Apply acupuncture and moxibustion.

6.24.5 崩漏五方
6.24.5 Prescription for Uterine Bleeding V

〔组成〕 合阳、中都。
Points: Heyang(BL 55), Zhongdu(LR 6).

〔来源〕 《普济方》。
Source: Puji Fang (Prescriptions for Curing All People).

〔功效〕 活血止血。
Action: Activating blood circulation and stopping uterine bleeding.

〔主治〕 崩中、腹上下痛。
Indication: Metrorrhagia with abdominal pain.

〔用法〕 毫针刺之。
Application: Apply acupuncture with filiform needle.

6.24.6 崩漏六方
6.24.6 Prescription for Uterine Bleeding VI

〔组成〕 漏阴穴(内踝下5分)。
Point: Rouyinxue (0.5 cun below the lower border of the internal

malleolus).

〔来源〕 《千金翼方》。
Source: Qianjin Yi Fang (Supplement to Valuable Prescriptions).

〔功效〕 固涩止血。
Action: Strengthening the vessels and stopping bleeding.

〔主治〕 崩漏。
Indication: Metrostaxis.

〔用法〕 艾灸。
Application: Apply moxibustion.

6.24.7 崩漏七方
6.24.7 Prescription for Uterine Bleeding Ⅶ

〔组成〕 耳子宫、卵巢、内分泌、脑点。
Point: Auricular points: Uteus, Ovary, Endocrine, Brain.

〔来源〕 吴春芳验方。
Source: Experience of Wu Chunfang.

〔功效〕 调宫止血。
Action: Regulating the function of uterus and stopping the uterine bleeding.

〔主治〕 崩漏。
Indication: Uterine bleeding.

〔用法〕 贴压法。
Application: Apply point-pressing.

6.25 乳腺增生类方
6.25 Prescriptions for Hyperplasia of Mammary Gland

6.25.1 乳癖一方
6.25.1 Prescription for Hyperplasia of Mammarry Gland Ⅰ

〔组成〕 太冲,肿块局部。
Points: Taichong(LR 1), points around the nodules of breast.

〔来源〕 作者验方。
Source: Experience of Fu Wenbin.

〔功效〕 疏肝理气、活血消肿。
Action: Disperssing the stagnated liver energy, activating the circulation of blood.

〔主治〕 乳腺增生。
Indication: Hyperplasia of mammary gland.

〔用法〕 太冲用泻法,肿块局部中心刺一针,周围边缘上下左右各刺一针。
Appication: Apply reducing method in Taichong (LR 3), then puncture a filiform needle into the centre of the nodule and four filiform needles around the nodule.

6.25.2 乳癖二方
6.25.2 Prescription for Hyperplasia of Mammary Gland Ⅱ

〔组成〕 耳肝、胃、乳腺、内分泌。

Points: Eye acupuncture: Liver, Stomach, Mammary gland, Endocrine.

〔来源〕 张和媛验方。

Source: Experience of Zhang Heyuan.

〔功效〕 调肝胃,消肿散结。

Action: Regulating the function of liver and stomach and resolvoving the nodule.

〔主治〕 乳腺增生。

Indication: Hyperlasia of mammary gland.

〔用法〕 毫针刺法或压丸法。

Application: Apply filiform acupuncture or point-pressing.

6.25.3 乳癖三方

6.25.3 Prescription for Hyperplasia of Mammary Gland III

〔组成〕 ①屋翳、膻中、合谷②肩井、天宗、肝俞。

Points: (1). Wuyi(ST 15), Tangzhong(RN 12), Hegu(LI 4); (2). Jianjing(GB 2), Tianzong(SI 11), Ganshu(BL 18).

〔来源〕 郭诚杰验方。

Source: Guo Chenjie's experience.

〔功效〕 解郁通经,止痛散结。

Action: Releasing the stagnated energy, resolving the nodule and relieving pain.

〔主治〕 乳腺增生。

Indicagion: Hyperplasia of mammary gland.

〔用法〕 两组交替使用,用平补平泻法。

Application: Apply even method, two groups of points are used alternatively.

6.26 胎位不正类方
6.26 Prescription for Abnormal Fetal Position

6.26.1 胎位不正一方
6.26.1 Prescriptions for Abnormal Fetal Position Ⅰ

〔组成〕 至阴。
Point: Zhiyin(BL 67).
〔来源〕 王全仁《中国针灸》1986(3)。
Source: Wangquanren 1986(3) Chinese Acupuncture and Moxibustion.
〔功效〕 调气血顺胎气。
Action: Adjusting the abnormal fetal position.
〔主治〕 胎位不正。
Indication: Abnormal fetal position.
〔用法〕 针灸并用。
Application: Apply acupuncture and moxibustion.

6.26.2 胎位不正二方
6.26.2 Prescription for Abnormal Fetal Position Ⅱ

〔组成〕 耳交感、子宫、皮质下、肝、脾、腹。
Points: Auricular point: Sympathetic nerve, Uterus, Subcortex, Liver, Spleen., Abdomen.
〔来源〕 秦广凤等《江苏中医》1986(8)。

Source: Qin Guangfeng etc. 1986(8) Jiangsu Journal of TCM.

〔功效〕 调气顺胎。

Action: Adjusting the abnormal fetal position.

〔主治〕 胎位不正。

Indication: Abnormal fetal positon.

〔用法〕 王不留行籽压贴法。

Application: Apply point-pressing with vaccaria seeds.

6.27 遗尿类方
6.27 Prescriptions for Enuresis

6.27.1 遗尿一方
6.27.1 Prescription for Enuresis I

〔组成〕 百会、关元、肾俞、次髎。

Points: Baihui(DU 20), Guanyuan(RN 4), Shenshu(BL 23), Ciliao(BL 32).

〔来源〕 喻喜春验方。

Source: Experience of Yu Xichun.

〔功效〕 调肾约束膀胱。

Action: Regulating the function of kidney and strengthening the urinary bladder.

〔主治〕 遗尿。

Indication: Enuresis.

〔用法〕 三棱针刺络。

Application: Apply spot prickling with three-edged needle.

6.27.2 遗尿二方
6.27.2 Prescription for Enuresis Ⅱ

〔组成〕 眼针肾区、下焦区。
Point: Eye acupuncture: Kidney and Lower burner areas.

〔来源〕 彭静山教授验方。
Source: Experience of Peng Jingshan.

〔功效〕 补肾调下元。
Action: Replenishing the kidney and regulating the function of lower burner.

〔主治〕 遗尿。
Indication: Enuresis.

〔用法〕 毫针刺之。
Application: Filiform needle acupuncture.

6.27.3 遗尿三方
6.27.3 Prescription for Enuresis Ⅲ

〔组成〕 足运感区(头皮针)。
Point: Scalp Acupuncture: Leg motor-sensory area.

〔来源〕 焦顺发验方。
Source: Experience of Jiao Sunfa.

〔功效〕 调理大脑皮质。
Action: Adjusting the function of cerebral cortex.

〔主治〕 小儿夜尿症。
Indicatipn: Nocturnal enuresis in children.

〔用法〕 毫针针刺。
Application: Filiform needle acupuncture.

6.27.4 遗尿四方
6.27.4 Prescription for Enuresis IV

〔组成〕 关元、三阴交。
Points: Guanyuan(RN 4), Sanyinjiao(SP 6).

〔来源〕 张唐法验方。
Source: Experience of Zhang Tangfa.

〔功效〕 补肾充下元。
Action: Replenishing Kidney.

〔主治〕 小儿夜尿。
Indication: Nocturnal enuresis in children.

〔用法〕 揿针埋入法。
Application: Embed the thumbtack intradermal needle.

6.27.5 遗尿五方
6.27.5 Prescription for Enuresis V

〔组成〕 百会、关元、三阴交、命门。
Points: Baihui(DU 20), Guanyuan(RN 4), Sanyinjiao(SP 6), Mingmen(DU 4).

〔来源〕 作者验方。
Source: Experience of authors.

〔功效〕 补肾培元,约束膀胱。
Action: Strengthening the function of urinary bladder and kidney.

〔主治〕 遗尿。
Indication: Enuresis.

〔用法〕 百会、关元、三阴交用补法,命门、关元用艾灸。
Application: Apply reinforcing in DU 20, RN 4 and SP 6; then

moxibustion in DU 4 and RN 4.

6.27.6 遗尿六方
6.27.6 Prescription for Enuresis Ⅵ

〔组成〕 箕门。
Point: Qimen(SP 11).
〔来源〕 杨日和《北京中医》1988(6)。
Source: Yang Rihe 1988(6) Beijing Journal of TCM.
〔功效〕 调下元,止遗尿。
Action: Tonifying the Kidney and rectifying uresis.
〔主治〕 遗尿
Indication: Enuresis.
〔用法〕 毫针针刺,补法。
Application: Apply reinforcing method with filiform needle.

6.28 牙痛类方
6.28 Prescriptions for Toothache

6.28.1 牙痛一方
6.28.1 Prescription for Toothache Ⅰ

〔组成〕 承浆、风府。
Points: Chengjang(RN 24), Fengfu(DU 16).
〔来源〕 《针方六集》。
Source: Zhenfang Liu Ji (Six Chapters of Acupuncture Prescriptions).

〔功效〕 祛风止痛
Action: Dispelling the wind and relieving toothache.
〔主治〕 牙痛。
Indication: Toothache.
〔用法〕 毫针针刺。
Application: Filiform needle acupuncture.

6.28.2 牙痛二方
6.28.2 Prescription for Toothache Ⅱ

〔组成〕 翳风。
Point: Yifeng(SJ 17).
〔来源〕 彭静山验方。
Source: Experience of Prof. PengJingshan.
〔功效〕 清热止痛。
Action: Clearing off heat and relieving toothache.
〔主治〕 牙痛。
Indication: Toothache.
〔用法〕 毫针针刺。
Application: Filiform needle acupuncture.

6.28.3 牙痛三方
6.28.3 Prescription for Toothache Ⅲ

〔组成〕 太阳。
Point: Taiyang(EX-HN 15).
〔来源〕 陈克勤验方。
Source: Experience of Chen Keqin.
〔功效〕 消炎止痛。

Action: Anti-inflammation and relieving toothache.

〔主治〕 牙痛。
Indication: Toothache.

〔用法〕 毫针泻法。
Application: Apply reducing method with filiform needle.

6.28.4 牙痛四方
6.28.4 Prescription for Toothache IV

〔组成〕 内踝尖。
Point: The apex of internal malleolus.

〔来源〕 《景岳全书》。
Source: Jing Yue Quan Shu (Jingyue's Complete Books).

〔功效〕 镇痛。
Action: relieving toothache.

〔主治〕 止牙痛。
Indication: Toothache.

〔用法〕 艾灸。
Application: Moxibustion.

6.28.5 牙痛五方
6.28.5 Prescription for Toothache V

〔组成〕 耳门、丝竹空。
Points: Ermen (SJ 21), Cizhukong (SJ 23).

〔来源〕 《百证赋》。
Source: Bai Zhen Fu (The Poems about the Acupuncture Treatment of Syndromes).

〔功效〕 清热消肿止痛。

Action: Clearing off the heat ,eliminating the swollen gums and relieving toothache.

〔主治〕 牙疼。

Indication: Toothache.

〔用法〕 毫针泻法。

Application: Apply reducing method with filiform needle.

6.29 咽喉肿痛类方
6.29 Prescriptions for Laryngopharyngitis

6.29.1 咽喉一方
6.29.1 Prescription for Laryngopharyngitis I

〔组成〕 少商、少冲。

Points: Shaoshang(LU 11), Shaochong(HT 9).

〔来源〕 《重楼玉钥》。

Source: Chong Lou Yu Yao (The Jade Key of Medical Mansion).

〔功效〕 清热利咽。

Action: Clearing off the heat and benefiting the throat.

〔主治〕 扁桃腺炎。

Indication: Tonsillitis.

〔用法〕 三棱针刺出血。

Application: Apply blood-letting with three-edged needle.

6.29.2 咽喉二方
6.29.2 Prescription for Laryngopharyngitis II

〔组成〕 然谷。
Point: Rangu(KI 2).
〔来源〕 《内经》。
Source: Neijing.
〔功效〕 清热养阴利咽。
Action: Clearing off the heat, nourishing the Yin and benefiting the throat.
〔主治〕 咽喉肿痛。
Indication: Sore and swollen throat.
〔用法〕 三棱针刺出血。
Application: Apply blood-letting with three-edged needle.

6.29.3 咽喉三方
6.29.3 Prescription for Laryngopharyngitis III

〔组成〕 列缺、照海。
Points: Lieque(LU 7), Zhaohai(LI 6).
〔来源〕 作者验方。
Source: Experience of authors.
〔功效〕 养阴润肺。
Action: Nourishing the Yin in the lungs.
〔主治〕 慢性咽炎。
Indication: Chronic pharyngitis.
〔用法〕 补照海,泻列缺。
Application: Apply reinforcing method in KI 6 and reducing in LU

7.

6.29.4 咽喉四方
6.29.4 Prescription for Laryngopharyngitis Ⅳ

〔组成〕 大椎。
Point：Dazhui(DU 14).
〔来源〕 喻喜春验方。
Source：Experience of Yu Xichung.
〔功效〕 清热泻火,消肿止痛。
Action：Clear off the heat and fire , eliminating the swelling and and relieving sore throat.
〔主治〕 急性扁桃体炎。
Indication：Acute tonsillitis.
〔用法〕 三棱针点刺3下加拔罐。
Application：Apply spot prickling three times in the point , then cupping.

6.30 痤疮类方
6.30 Prescriptions for Acne

6.30.1 痤疮一方
6.30.1 Prescripition for Acne Ⅰ

〔组成〕 拳尖(位于第三掌骨小头高点)。
Point：Quanjian(The apex of the fist apex of the small head of third metacarpal bone).

〔来源〕《针灸秘验》。
Source: Zhenjiu Mi Yan (Secret Experience of Acupuncture).

〔功效〕 活血消肿。
Action: Activating the circulation of blood and eliminating the swelling.

〔主治〕 痤疮。
Indication: Acne.

〔用法〕 艾灸。
Application: Moxibustion.

6.30.2 痤疮二方
6.30.2 Prescription for Acne Ⅱ

〔组成〕 ①大椎、肺俞;②耳心、肺、内分泌,神门。
Points: (1) Dazhui (DU 14), Feishu (BL 13) (2). Auricular *Points*: Heart, Lungs, Endocrine and Shenmen.

〔来源〕 作者验方
Source: Experience of authors.

〔功效〕 清热消肿。
Action: Clearing off heat and eliminating the swelling.

〔主治〕 痤疮。
Indication: Acne.

〔用法〕 体针组用三棱针点刺加拔罐;耳穴用王不留行籽按压。
Application: Apply three-edged needle spot prickling in points of group (1); then, apply point-pressing in auricular points

6.31 痹证类方
6.31 Prescriptions for Bi-syndrome

6.31.1 痹证 1 方
6.31.1 Prescription for Bi-syndrome

〔组成〕 膈俞、脾俞、膀胱俞。
Points: Geshu(BL 17), Pishu(BL 20), Pangguangshu(BL 28)
〔来源〕 司徒铃教授验方。
Source: Experience of Situ Ling.
〔功效〕 健脾祛湿,活血通络。
Action: Invigorating spleen and promoting diuresis, activating blood circulation and dredging the collaterals.
〔主治〕 周痹。
Indication: Dampness type Bi-syndrome, localized arthralgia with a heavy sensation.
〔用法〕 艾灸
Application: Moxibustion.

6.31.2 痹证 2 方
6.31.2 Prescription for Bi-syndrome II

〔组成〕 委中、四花、尺泽。
Points: Weizhong(BL 40), Four flowers *Points* (bilateral BL 17 and BL 19), Chize(LU 5).
〔来源〕 作者验方。

Source: Experience of authors.

〔功效〕 清热利湿,清肿止痛。

Action: clearing off the heat and dampness, eliminating the swelling of joint and relieving arthralgia.

〔主治〕 热痹。

Indication: Heat Bi-syndrome (Painful, reddish, and swollen joints).

〔用法〕 三棱针刺络加拔罐。

Application: Apply spot pricking then cupping.

6.31.3 痹证三方
6.31.3 Prescription for Bi-syndrome Ⅲ

〔组成〕 涌泉、昆仑。

Points: Yongquan(LI 1), Kunlun(BL 60).

〔来源〕 《内经》。

Source: Neijing.

〔功效〕 祛寒补肾。

Action: Dispelling the cold evil and tonifying the kidney.

〔主治〕 阴痹。

Indication: Yin type of Bi-syndrome.

〔用法〕 毫针刺之或三棱针刺出血。

Application: Apply filiform needle acupuncture or spot pricking with three-edged needle for blood-letting.

6.31.4 痹证四方
6.31.4 Prescription for Bi-syndrome Ⅳ

〔组成〕 三阳络、环跳。

Points: Sanyanglo(SJ 8), Huantiao(GB 30).

〔来源〕 欧阳伟验方。
Source:Experience of Euyang Wei.
〔功效〕 祛风湿,通经络。
Action:Dispelling the wind and cold,dredging collaterals.
〔主治〕 痹证。
Indication:Bi-syndrome.
〔用法〕 毫针针刺。
Application:Filiform needle acupuncture.

6.31.5 痹证五方
6.31.5 Prescription for Bi-syndrome V

〔组成〕 天枢、阴交、水分。
Points:Tianshu(ST 25),Yinjiao(RN 7),Shuifen(RN 9)
〔来源〕 张世雄《中国针灸》1990(3)。
Source:Zhang Shixong 1990(3) Chinese Acupuncture and moxibustion.
〔功效〕 祛风湿通络。
Action:Dispelling the wind and eliminating dampness,and dredging the collaterals.
〔主治〕 痹证。
Indication:Bi-syndrome.
〔用法〕 毫针针刺。
Applicatioln:Filiform needle acupuncture.

6.32 面肌痉挛类方
6.32 Prescriptions for Muscular Spasm of Face

6.32.1 痉挛一方
6.31.1 Prescription for Facial Muscle spasm Ⅰ

〔组成〕 四关、眼肝区。
Points:Four-gate Points(Bilateral LI 4 and LR 3)and Liver area in eye acupunctre.

〔来源〕 作者验方。
Source:Experience of authors.

〔功能〕 平肝熄风止痉。
Action:Calming the liver to inhibit the endogenous wind and relaxing the spasm.

〔主治〕 面肌痉挛。
Indication:Facial muscle spasm.

〔用法〕 毫针泻法。
Application:Apply reducing method with filiform needle.

6.32.2 痉挛二方
6.32.2 Prescription for Facial Muscle Spasm Ⅱ

〔组成〕 印堂、人中、承浆、抽动点。
Pionts:Yintang(EX-HN 3),Renzhong(RN 26),Chengjiang(RN 24),Spas *Points*;.

〔来源〕 梁清湖验方

Source: Experience of Liang Qinhu.

〔功效〕 祛风止痉。

Action: Dispelling the wind and relieving spasm.

〔主治〕 面肌痉挛。

Indication: Facial muscle spasm.

〔用法〕 先在印堂、人中、承浆从上而下浅刺,再在抽动点向跳动延伸方向透刺 1-2 寸。

Application: Apply shallow puncture in Yintang, Renzhong and Chengjiang; then apply penetrating puncture, inserting the needle in spastic points, penetrating 1-2 cun along the passage of spastic muscle.

6.32.3 痉挛三方
6.32.3 Prescription for Faceial Muscle Spasm Ⅲ

〔组成〕 发痉点

Point: Spastic point.

〔来源〕 《针灸秘验》。

Source: Exerience of Peng Jingshan.

〔功效〕 熄风止痉。

Action: Inhibiting wind and controlling spasm.

〔主治〕 面肌痉挛。

Indication: Facial muscle spasm.

〔用法〕 先用梅花针轻叩患侧面,至某部位一触即发痉,此部为发痉点,即在其处埋揿针,三日后去针,反复多次。

Application: Applying light plum blossom needling on the affected face, then the attack of facial muscle spasm will be induced. Find out the most obvious spastic points. Embed the intradermal needle in that point and retain it for three days. Repeat the treatment a couple of times。

6.33 咳嗽类方
6.33 Prescription for Cough

6.33.1 咳嗽一方
6.33.1 Prescription for Cough Ⅰ

〔组成〕 天突、肺俞。
Points:Tiantu(RN 22),Feishu(BL 13)。
〔来源〕 《金匮钩玄》。
Source:Jin Gui Gu Xuan (The Description of the Gist of Golden Chamber Synopsis)。
〔功效〕 祛痰温肺止咳。
Action:Warming the lungs, eliminating the sputum and relieving cough.
〔主治〕 寒痰咳嗽。
Indication:Cough due to cold sputum accumulation.
〔用法〕 直接灸。
Application:Direct moxibustion.

6.33.2 咳嗽二方
6.33.2 Prescription For Cough Ⅱ

〔组成〕 眼针上焦、肺区。
Points:Eye acupuncture:Upper burner and Lungs areas.
〔来源〕 作者验方。

Source: Experience of authors.

〔功效〕 宣肺止咳。

Action: Releasing the inhibited lung energy.

〔主治〕 咳嗽频频。

Indication: Cough frequently

〔用法〕 毫针针刺。

Application: Apply filiform needle puncture.

6.33.3 咳嗽三方
6.33.3 Prescription for Cough Ⅲ

〔组成〕 肺俞、膻中、尺泽、太溪。

Points: Feishu (BL 13), Tangzhong (RN 17), Chize (LU 5), Taixi (KI 3).

〔来源〕 《神灸经纶》。

Source: Shen Jiu Jing Lun (The Protocol of Miracullous Moxibustion).

〔功效〕 清泻肺热，肃肺止咳。

Action: Clearing away heat evil and releasing inhibited energy in the lungs, relieving cough.

〔主治〕 肺热咳嗽。

Indication: Cough due to heat evil in the lungs.

〔用法〕 毫针泻法。

Application: Apply reducing method with filiform needle.

6.34 感冒类方
6.34 Prescriptions for Common Cold

6.34.1 感冒一方
6.34.1 Prescription for Common cold I

〔组成〕 大椎。
Point: Dazhui(DU 14)
〔来源〕 曹仁和《江苏中医》1986(5)。
Source: Cao Renhe 1986(5) Jiangsu Journal of TCM.
〔功效〕 祛风寒解表。
Action: Dispelling the wind cold evil.
〔主治〕 流感（风寒型）。
Indication: Influenza differentiated as type wind-cold in TCM.
〔用法〕 艾灸。
Application: Moxibustion.

6.34.2 感冒二方
6.34.2 Prescription for Common Cold II

〔组成〕 身柱。
Point: Shenzhu(DU 12).
〔来源〕 彭静山验方。
Source: Experience of Peng Jingshan.
〔功效〕 强身固表祛风。
Action: Strengthening the exterior and dispelling the wind evil.

〔主治〕 经常感冒。

Indication: for the prevention of common cold.

〔用法〕 深刺1.5寸。

Application: Puncture the needle with a depth of 1.5 cun.

6.34.3 感冒三方
6.34.3 Prescription for Common Cold III

〔组成〕 天柱、合谷、背俞。

Points: Tianzhu(BL 10), Hegu(LI 4), Back-shu *points*:.

〔来源〕 作者验方。

Source: Experience of authors.

〔功效〕 祛风解表。

Action: Dispelling the wind and relieving superficial syndrome.

〔主治〕 感冒。

Indication: Common cold.

〔用法〕 先毫针泻天柱、合谷,后在背俞拔罐。

Application: Apply reducing method in Tianzhu and Hegu with filiform needles, then cupping in the Back-shu Points.

6.34.4 感冒四方
6.34.4 Prescription for Common Cold IV

〔组成〕 中渚。

Point: Zhongzhu(SJ 3).

〔来源〕 申健《河南中医》1988(4)。

Source: Shen Jian 1989(4) Henan Journal of TCM.

〔功效〕 祛风解表。

Action: Dispelling the wind evil and relieving the superficial syndrome.

〔主治〕 感冒。

Indication: Common cold.

〔用法〕 毫针泻法。

Application: Apply reducing method with filiform needle.

6.35 肥胖类方
6.35 Prescriptions for Obesity

6.35.1 肥胖一方
6.35.1 Prescription for Obesity Ⅰ

〔组成〕 梁丘、公孙。

Points: Liangqiu(ST 34), Gongsun(SP 4).

〔来源〕 雷振萍《中医杂志》1987(5)。

Source: Le Zhenpin 1987(5) Journal of TCM.

〔功效〕 理脾减肥。

Action: Regulating the function of spleen and losing weight.

〔主治〕 肥胖症。

Indication: Simple obesity.

〔用法〕 先用电针,后埋皮内针。

Application: Apply electric acupuncture and embed the intradermal needle.

6.35.2 肥胖二方
6.35.2 Prescription for obesity Ⅱ

〔组成〕 耳穴三焦、肺、内分泌。
Points:Auricular pionts:Triple burner,Lungs,and Endocrine area.

〔来源〕 李士杰《中国针灸》1986(3)。
Source:LiSijie 1986(3) Chinese Acupuncture and Moxibustion.

〔功效〕 调理三焦。
Action:Regulation the function of triple burner.

〔主治〕 肥胖症。
Indication:Simple obesity.

〔用法〕 耳穴埋揿针。
Application:Embed intradermal needle in the points.

6.35.3 肥胖三方
6.35.3 Prescription for Obesity Ⅲ

〔组成〕 ①百会、内关、梁丘、足三里、关元;②耳穴胃、脾、肺。
Points:(1). Baihui(DU 20),Neiguang(PC 6),Liang Qiu(ST 34),Zusanli(ST 36) Guanyuan(RN 4)(2). Auricular points:Stomach, Lungs and Spleen.

〔来源〕 梁清湖验方。
Source:Liang Qinhu's experience

〔功效〕 祛痰湿降脂减肥。
Action:Eliminating phlegm and dampness ,lowering the blood-lipid and weight.

〔主治〕 单纯性肥胖症。
Indication: Simple obesity.

〔用法〕 毫针泻法,耳穴用穴位压迫法。
Application:Apply reducing method with filiform needle in points of group (1)and point-pressing in auricular points.

6.35.4 肥胖四方
6.35.4 Prescription for Obesity Ⅱ

〔组成〕 耳穴三焦、肺、内分泌。
Points:Auricular Points,Triple burner ,Lungs and Endocrine.
〔来源〕 李士杰《中国针灸》1986(3)。
Source:Li Shijie 1986(3) Chinese Acupuncture and Moxibustion.
〔功效〕 调理三焦减肥。
Action:Regulating the function of triple burner to lower weight.
〔主治〕 单纯肥胖症。
Indication:Simple Obesity.
〔用法〕 掀针埋藏法。
Application:Apply point-pressing or embed intradermal needle.

6.36 戒毒、戒烟、戒酒类方
6.36 Prescriptions for Quitting Smoking,the Treatment of Drug-addict and Alcohol Dependence.

6.36.1 戒毒方
6.36.1 Prescription for the Treatment of Drug Dependence

〔组成〕 ①内关、三阴交、百会;②耳:心、肺、神门、皮质下。

Points: (1). Neiguang(PC 6), Sanyinjiao(SP 6), Baihui(DU 20) (2). Auricular ooints: Heart, Shenmen, Lungs and Subcortex.

〔来源〕 作者验方。
Source: Experience of Fu Wenbin.
〔功效〕 调心肺戒毒瘾。
Action: Regulating the function of heart and lungs.
〔主治〕 吸毒戒断症状。
Indication: Symptoms of drug dependence.
〔用法〕 先用毫针泻体穴,再在耳穴埋揿针。
Application: Apply the reducing method in the points of group(1) and embed the intradermal needle in auricular points.

6.36.2 戒烟方
6.36.2 Prescription for Quitting Smoking

〔组成〕 耳穴口、肺、神门。
Points: Auricular points: Mouth, Lungs and Shenmen.
〔来源〕 方幼安验方。
Source: Fang youan's experience.
〔功效〕 戒烟。
Action: Quitting cigarette smoking.
〔主治〕 烟瘾者。
Indication: Smoking habit.
〔用法〕 毫针重刺激。
Application: Apply intense stimulation with filiform needle.

6.36.3 戒酒方
6.36.3 Prescription for Treatment of Alcohol Dependence

〔组成〕 耳神门、皮质下、心、胃、内分泌、咽喉。

Points: Shenmen, Subcortex, Heart, Stomach and Endocrine Larynx and Pharynx.

〔来源〕 孙申田《中医杂志》1987(3)。

Source: Sun Shentian 1987(3) Journal of TCM.

〔功效〕 调心胃戒酒。

Action: Regulating the function of Heart and Stomach, and withdrawing alcohol.

〔主治〕 酒瘾。

Indication: Alcohol addict.

〔用法〕 每次选2~4穴,埋揿针或王不留行籽。

Application: Apply points-pressing or embed intradermal needle at 2-4 points in each treatment.

6.37 瘾疹类方
6.37 Prescriptions for Urticaria

6.37.1 瘾疹一方
6.37.1 Prescription for Urticaria I

〔组成〕 曲池、绝骨、委中。

Points: Quchi(LI 11), Juegu(GB 39), Weizhong(BL 40).

〔来源〕 《扁鹊神应针灸玉龙经》。
Source: Yu Long Jing (The Classic of Jade Dragon).

〔功效〕 祛风去毒,活血止痒。
Action: Dispelling wind, detoxication, activating the blood circualtion and relieving the itching of skin.

〔主治〕 瘾疹。
Indication: Urticaria.

〔用法〕 先泻曲池、绝骨,委中放血。后直接灸曲池、绝骨。
Application: Apply reducing in LI 11 and GB 39, blood-letting in GB 40; apply the direct moxibustion in LI11 and GB 39.

6.37.2 瘾疹二方
6.37.2 Prescription for Urticaria II

〔组成〕 大椎、肺俞、天突、鸠尾。
Pionts: Dazhui (DU 14), Feishu (BL 13), Tiantu (RN 22) Jiuwei (KRN 15).

〔来源〕 司徒铃验方。
Source: Experience of Situ Ling.

〔功效〕 祛风活血固卫。
Action: Dispelling the wind, activatng blood circulation and strengthening the exterior of body.

〔主治〕 荨麻疹(慢性)。
Indication: Chronic urticaria.

〔用法〕 挑治,每周一次。
Application: Apply pricking therapy in the points, once a week.

6.37.3 瘾疹三方
6.37.3 Prescription for Urticaria Ⅲ

〔组成〕 委中、膈俞、尺泽、大椎。
Pionts: Weizhong(BL 40), Geshu(BL 17), chize(LU 5), Dazhui(DU 14).

〔来源〕 作者验方。
Source: Experience of authors.

〔功效〕 祛风活血。
Action: Dispelling the wind and activating the blood circulation.

〔主治〕 荨麻疹。
Indication: Urticaria.

〔用法〕 刺络放血。
Application: Apply the spot pricking for blood-letting.

6.37.4 瘾疹四方
6.37.4 Prescription for Urticaria Ⅳ

〔组成〕 足三里、曲池、关元、中脘、天枢、肺俞、血海。
Pionts: Zusanli(ST 36), Quchi(LI 11), Guanyuan(RN 12), Tianshu(ST 25), Feishu(BL 13), Xuehai(SP 10).

〔来源〕 乔正中验方。
Source: Experience of Qiao Zhenzhong.

〔功效〕 和气血通经络。
Action: Regulating the circulation of Qi and blood, dredging the collaterals.

〔主治〕 荨麻疹。
Indication: Urticaria.

〔用法〕 火针点刺。
Application:Apply spot pricking with a burning needle.

6.37.5 瘾疹五方
6.37.5 Prescription for Urticaria V

〔组成〕 神阙。
Point :Shenjue(RN 8).
〔来源〕 刘天峰《中医杂志》1986(12)。
Source:Experience of Liu Tianfeng,1986(12) Journal of TCM.
〔功效〕 祛风消疹。
Action:Dispelling the wind and ellminating rashes.
〔主治〕 急慢性荨麻疹。
Indication:Urticaria.
〔用法〕 拔罐。
Application:Cupping.

6.37.6 瘾疹六方
6.37.6 Prescription for Urticaria VI

〔组成〕 耳穴肺、荨麻疹点、枕、肾上腺、内分泌。
Pionts:Lungs,Urticaria points,Occiput,Adrenal,Endocrine.
〔来源〕 李志明《耳穴诊治法》。
Source:Erxue Zhen Zi Fa (The Auricular Points Diagnostic and Therapy).
〔功效〕 疏风止痒,抗过敏。
Action:Dispelling the wind and stopping the itching of skin.
〔主治〕 荨麻疹。
Indication:Urticaria.

〔用法〕 毫针针刺或耳穴贴药籽法。

Application：Apply filiform needle acupuncture or points-pressing.

6.38 痔疮类方
6.38 Prescriptions for Hemorrhoid

6.38.1 痔疮一方
6.38.1 Prescription for Hemorrhoid I

〔组成〕 二白。

Point：Erbai(EX-UE2).

〔来源〕 《玉龙经》。

Source：Yu Long Jing (The Classic of Jade Dragon).

〔功效〕 祛湿行瘀止血。

Action：Eliminating the dampness and removing the blood stasis to stop bleeding.

〔主治〕 痔疮。

Indication：Hemorrhoid.

〔用法〕 针灸均可。

Application：Acupuncture or moxibustion.

6.38.2 痔疮二方
6.38.2 Prescription for Hemorrhoid II

〔组成〕 长强、承山。

Points：Changqiang(DU 1), Chengshan(BL 57).

〔来源〕 《玉龙歌》。

Source: Yu Long jing (Classis of Jade Dragon).

〔功效〕 清热利湿,止血镇痛。

Action: Eliminating heat and dampness, stopping bleeding and relieving pain.

〔主治〕 痔疮。

Indication: Hemorrhoid.

〔用法〕 毫针泻法。

Application: Apply reducing method with filiform needle.

6.38.3 痔疮三方
6.38.3 Prescription for Hemorrhoid Ⅲ

〔组成〕 攒竹。

Point: Zanzhu (BL 2).

〔来源〕 《针灸甲乙经》。

Source: Zhen Jiu Ja Yi Jing (AB Classic of Acupuncture and Moxibustion)

〔功效〕 行血止痛。

Action: Activating the blood circulation and relieving pain.

〔主治〕 痔疮疼痛。

Indication: Pain in hemorrhoid.

〔用法〕 毫针针刺。

Application: Apply reducing method with filiform needle.

6.38.4 痔疮四方
6.38.4 Prescription for Hemorrhoid Ⅳ

〔组成〕 大肠俞、长强。

Pionts: Dachangshu (BL 25), Changqiang (DU 11).

〔来源〕 作者验方。

Source: Experience of authors.

〔功效〕 活血消肿止痛。

Action: Activating the blood circulation, resolving the swelling and relieving pain.

〔主治〕 痔疮肿痛。

Indication: Swollen and painful hemorrhoid.

〔用法〕 针刺或针挑。

Application: Apply acupuncture or pricking therapy.

6.39 保健类方
6.39 Prescriptions for Health Preserving

6.39.1 保健一方
6.39.1 Prescription for Health Preserving I

〔组成〕 足三里

Point: Zusanli(ST 36).

〔来源〕 《医说》。

Source: Yi Shou(The Explantion of Medicine).

〔功效〕 健脾延年益寿。

Action: Replenishing the spleen and preserving the health.

〔主治〕 脾虚食欲不振、消化不良,未老先衰。

Idication: Poor appetite, indigestion due to spleen deficiency, premature aging.

〔用法〕 疤痕灸

Application: Apply scarring moxibustion.

6.39.2 保健二方
6.39.2 Prsecription for Health Preserving II

〔组成〕 关元、命门。
Points: Guanyuan(RN 4), Mingmen(DU 4).

〔来源〕《扁鹊心书》。
Source: Bianque Xion Shu (The Gist of Bianque's Medical Thought).

〔功效〕 益真元,健体轻身.
Action: Replenishing kidney essence and preserving health

〔主治〕 肾虚体弱,经常腰痛,夜尿多,防衰老。
Idication: Low back pain, profuse nocturnal urine, premature aging.

〔用法〕 直接灸。
Application: Direct moxibustion.

6.39.3 保健三方
6.39.3 Prescription for Health Preserving III

〔组成〕 足三里、绝骨。
Points: Zusanli(ST 36), Juegu(GB 39).

〔来源〕《针灸资生经》。
Source: Zhenjiu Zhi Sheng Jing (The Classic of Acupuncture and Moxibustion for the Benefit of All People).

〔功效〕 预防中风。
Action: Preventing "wind-stroke"

〔主治〕 中风先兆。

Idication: Premonitory symptoms of wind strock.

〔用法〕 艾灸。

Application: Moxibustion.

6.40 胆绞痛类方
6.40 Prescriptions for Biliary Colic

6.40.1 胆绞痛一方
6.40.1 Prescription for Biliary Colic Ⅰ

〔组成〕 眼针肝、胆、中焦。

Points: Eye acupuncture: Liver, Gallbladder and Middle burner areas.

〔来源〕 王济华等《中国针灸》1989(2)。

Source: Wang Jihua etal, 1989(2) Chinese Acupuncture and Moxibustion.

〔功效〕 疏肝利胆,镇痛。

Action: Disperssing the stagnated liver Qi and promoting the Qi movement of the gallbladder, relieving the colic.

〔主治〕 胆绞痛。

Indication: Biliary colic.

〔用法〕 毫针针刺。

Application: Filiform needle acupuncture.

6.40.2 胆绞痛二方
6.40.2 Prescription for Biliary Colic Ⅱ

〔组成〕 鸠尾、膻中、阳陵泉。
Points: Jiuwei (RN 15), Tangzhoug (RN 17), Yanglingquan (GB 34).

〔来源〕 觉正祥等《中西医结合杂志》1989(3)。
Source: Jue Zhengxiang 1989(3) Journal of Combination of TCM and Western Medicine.

〔功效〕 理气利胆止痛。
Action: Activating the circulation of Qi in gallbladder and relieving pain.

〔主治〕 胆绞痛。
Idication: Biliary colic.

〔用法〕 鸠尾透膻中,阳陵泉用泻法。
Application: Apply penetrating puncture from RN 15 to RN 17, and reducing in GB 34.

6.40.3 胆绞痛三方
6.40.3 Prescription for Biliary Colic Ⅲ

〔组成〕 神阙。
Points: Shenjue (RN 8).

〔来源〕 喻峰等《河南中医杂志》1987(6)。
Source: Yu Feng etc. 1987(6) Henan Journal of TCM.

〔功效〕 温经散寒止痛。
Action: Warming the meridians and dispelling the cold, relieving pain.

〔主治〕 胆绞痛。
Idication：Biliary colic.

〔用法〕 艾灸。
Application：Moxibustion.

6.41 肾绞痛类方
6.41 Prescriptions for The Renal Colic

6.41.1 肾绞痛一方
6.41.1 Prescription for The Renal Colic Ⅰ

〔组成〕 足三里、三阴交、肾俞。
Points：Zusanli(ST 36). Sanyinjiao(SP 6), Shenshu(BL 23).

〔来源〕 区向阳《中国针灸》1989(4)。
Source：Qu Xiangyang 1989(4) Chinese Acupuncture and Moxibustion

〔功效〕 理气镇痛。
Action：Activating Qi circulation and relieving pain.

〔主治〕 肾绞痛。
Idication：Renal colic.

〔用法〕 毫针泻法。
Application：Apply reducing method with filiform needle.

6.41.2 肾绞痛二方
6.41.2 Prescription for The Renal Colic Ⅱ

〔组成〕 踝腕针,穴位在内、外踝最高点上方3横指水平取穴,1穴在内侧面中央靠近胫骨内侧缘,另1穴在外侧面中央腓骨嵴与邻近肌腱所形成的浅沟内。

Points:Wrist-ankle acupuncture

Points 1:beside the medial border of tibia, at the level of 3 fingers breadth above the apex of internal mallelous.

Point 2:in the depression between the fibula process and tendons at the level of 3-fingers breadth above the apex of external mallelous

〔来源〕 张先清《中国针灸》1987(5)。

Source:Zhang Xiantiao 1987(5) Chinese Acupuncture and Moxibustion.

〔功效〕 调气止痛。

Action:Regulating the circulation of Qi and relieving the pain.

〔主治〕 肾绞痛。

Indication:Renal colic.

〔用法〕 取患侧,毫针向上斜刺。

Application:Select the points at the affected side (renal colic), apply the filiform needle acupuncture with an upward-oblique insertion.

6.41.3 肾绞痛三方

6.41.3 Prescription for The Renal Colic Ⅲ

〔组成〕 眼针肾区。

Point:Eye acupuncture:Kidney area.

〔来源〕 作者验方。

Source:Experience of authors.

〔功效〕 调肾镇痛。

Action:Regulating the function of kidney and relieving the renal colic.

〔主治〕 肾绞痛。
Indication: Renal colic.
〔用法〕 毫针针刺。
Application: Filiform needle acupuncture.

6.42 三叉神经痛类方
6.42 Prescriptions for Trigeminal Neuralgia

6.42.1 三叉神经痛一方
6.42.1 Prescription for Trigeminal Neuralgia Ⅰ

〔组成〕 人迎。
Point: Renying(ST 9).
〔来源〕 程正云等《陕西中医》1985(2)。
Source: Cheng Zhengyun 1985(2) Sangxi Journal of TCM.
〔功效〕 清胃止痛。
Action: Clearing away heat in the stomach meridian and relieving facial pain.
〔主治〕 三叉神经痛。
Indication: Trigeminal neuralgia.
〔用法〕 毫针针刺。
Application: Apply filiform needle acupucnture.

6.42.2 三叉神经痛二方
6.42.2 Prescription for Trigeminal Neuralgia Ⅱ

〔组成〕 鱼腰、四白、下关、夹承浆。
Points: Yuyao (EX-HN4), Sibai (ST 2), Xiaguang (ST 7),

Jachengjiang (1 cun beside the RN 24).

〔来源〕 葛书翰等《中医杂志》1987(6)。

Source: Ge Shuhan etc. 1987(6) Journal of TCM.

〔功效〕 疏通经络气血。

Action: Activating the circulation of blood and Qi in the meridian and collateral.

〔主治〕 三叉神经痛。

Idication: Trigeminal neuralgia.

〔用法〕 第1支痛取鱼腰,第2支痛取四白,第3支痛取下关或配夹承浆,均泻法。

Application: If the first branch of trigeminal nerve is involved, puncture the Yuyao (EX-HN4); second branch, puncture Sibai; third branch, or second and third involved together, puncture the Xiaguan point only, or in combination with Jiachengjiang.

6.43 内耳眩晕类方
6.43 Prescriptions for Auditory Vertigo

6.43.1 内耳眩晕一方
6.43.1 Prescription for Auditory Vertigo I

〔组成〕 太冲左、丰隆右、听宫双、三阴交右、合谷(耳鸣侧)、内关左。

Points: Left Taichong (LR 3), right Fenglong (SJ 40), bilateral Tinggong (SJ 19), right Sanyinjiao (SP 6), Hegu (LI 4) of affected side, left Neiguang (PC 6).

〔来源〕 杨秀《中国针灸》1984(2)。

Source: Yang Xiu 1984(2) Chinaese Acupuncture and Moxibustion.

〔功效〕 平肝熄风,养血安神。

Action: Calming the hyperactivity of liver Yang to inhibit the endogenous wind, nourishing the blood and benefiting the mind.

〔主治〕 内耳眩晕。

Idication: Auditory vertigo.

〔用法〕 太冲、丰隆、听宫用平补平泻,三阴交补法,合谷、内关均用泻。

Application: Apply even method in points Taichong, Fenglong, and Tinggong, reinforcing in point Sanyinjiao; and reducing in points Hegu and Neiguang.

6.43.2 内耳眩晕二方
6.43.2 Prescription for Auditory Vertigo II

〔组成〕 百会。

Point: Baihui (DU 20).

〔来源〕 司徒铃验方。

Source: Experience of Situ Ling.

〔功效〕 祛痰浊,平肝定晕。

Action: Eliminating the phlegm and turbid fluid, calming down liver Yang.

〔主治〕 内耳性眩晕。

Indication: Auditory vertigo.

〔用法〕 压灸。

Application: Direct moxibustion with moxa cone, then pressing and extingusihing the cone with a moxa stick to let warm sensation penetrate downwards.

6.44 足跟痛类方
6.44 Prescriptions for Heel Pain

6.44.1 足跟痛一方
6.44.1 Prescription for Heel Pain Ⅰ

〔组成〕 大陵。
Point: Daling (PC 7).
〔来源〕 赵怀儒《河北中医》1985(4)。
Source: Zhao Huairu 1985(4) Hebai Journal of TCM.
〔功效〕 活血通络。
Action: Activating the circulation of blood and dredging the collaterals.
〔主治〕 跟骨骨刺痛。
Indication: Pain in heel due to spur.
〔用法〕 毫针平补平泻。
Application: Apply even method with filiform needle.

6.44.2 足跟痛二方
6.44.2 Prescription for Heel Pain Ⅱ

〔组成〕 风池。
Point: Fengchi (GB 20).
〔来源〕 赵下成《中医杂志》1986(11)。

Source: Zhao Xiachen 1986(11) Journal of TCM.

〔功效〕 祛风通经。

Action: Dispelling the wind and dredging the collaterals.

〔主治〕 足跟痛。

Action: Pain in heel.

〔用法〕 毫针针刺。

Application: Filiform needle acupuncture.

6.44.3 足跟痛三方
6.44.3 Prescription for Heel Pain Ⅲ

〔组成〕 合谷穴向后约1寸处。

Point: Point 1 cun above the Hegu(LI 4).

〔来源〕 梁焕之《中医杂志》1985(2)。

Source: Liang Huanzi 1985(2) Journal of TCM.

〔功效〕 通络止痛。

Action: Dredging the collaterals and relieving pain.

〔主治〕 足跟痛。

Indication: Pain in heel.

〔用法〕 毫针直刺。

Application: Filiform needle acupuncture.

6.45 颈椎病类方
6.45 Prescriptions for Cervical Spondylopathy

6.45.1 颈椎一方
6.45.1 Prescription for Cervical Spondylopathy Ⅰ

〔组成〕 颈 2~6 夹脊、养老。
Points:Yanglao(SI 6),Jiaji(EX-B 2,from 2ed to 6th cervical vertebra.

〔来源〕 林迎春《浙江中医》1987(2)。
Source:Ling Yingchun 1987(2) Zhejiang Journal of TCM.

〔功效〕 行气活血,祛湿通络。
Action:Activating the circulation of blood and Qi ,eliminating the dampness and dredging the collaterals.

〔主治〕 颈椎病。
Indication:Cervical spondylopathy.

〔用法〕 电针。
Application:Electric acupuncture.

6.45.2 颈椎二方
6.45.2 Prescription for Cervical Spondylopathy Ⅱ

〔组成〕 新设(在第三、四颈椎之间,旁开 1.5 寸)、大椎、肩外俞、膈俞。
Points:Xinse("Point newly developed",1.5 cun beside the middle line of the back,at the level of middle point between 3rd and 4th cervi-

cal vertebra),Dazhui(DU 14),Jianzhongshu(SI 14),Geshu(BL 17).

〔来源〕 作者验方。

Source:Experience of authors.

〔功效〕 活血祛瘀,通络止痛。

Action:Removing the blood stasis,dredging the collaterals and relieving pian.

〔主治〕 颈椎病。

Indication:Cervical spondylopathy.

〔用法〕 挑治。

Application:Pricking therapy.

6.45.3 颈椎三方

6.45.3 Prescription for Cervical Spondylopathy Ⅲ

〔组成〕 主(耳)穴:肺、肾、颈项;配穴:内分泌、交感、肩、枕、心、脾。

Points:Dominant Point: Kidney and Liver;Supplementary Points: Endocrine,Sympathetic nerve,Shoulder,Occiput,Heart,Spleen.

〔来源〕 潘纪华《陕西中医》1987(8)。

Source:Pan Jihua 1987(8) Shanxi Journal of TCM.

〔功效〕 调肝肾,利筋通络。

Indication:Cervical spondylopathy.

〔主治〕 颈椎病。

Action:Regulating the kidney and liver function ,dredging the collaterals and benefiting the tendons.

〔用法〕 用耳穴压丸法。以主耳穴为主。痛甚加神门、交感,骨赘控制不理想加内分泌,沉困无力加脾,后头痛加枕,背肩痛加肩,帮助复位加心、交感。

Application: Apply the point-pressing method in dominant points; for severe pain, plus Shenmen; for spur, Endocrine; for heavy sensation of body, Spleen; occipital headache, Occiput; for pain in shoulder and back, Shoulder points; for abnormal position of cervical vertebra, Heart and Sympathetic nerve points.

4.46 治癣类方
6.46 Prescriptions for The Treatment of Tinea

4.46.1 治癣一方
4.46.1 Prescription for The Treatment of Tinea Ⅰ

〔组成〕 绝骨、足三里、间使、解溪、委中。
Points: Juegu (GB 39), Zusanli (ST 36), Jianshi (PC 5) Jiexi (ST 41), Weizhong (BL 40).

〔来源〕 《针灸集成》。
Source: Zhen Jiu Ji Cheng (Collection of Acupuncture and Moxibustion Works).

〔功效〕 祛风活血润燥。
Action: Dispelling wind, activating the blood circulation, moisturizing the dryness.

〔主治〕 顽癣。
Indication: Intractable tinea.

〔用法〕 针灸均可。
Application: Acupuncture and moxibustion.

6.46.2 治癣二方
6.46.2 Prescription for The Treatment of Tinea

〔组成〕 玉枕。
Point:YuZhen(BL 9).
〔来源〕 宋君惠《中国针灸》1985(3)。
Source:Song Junhui 1985(3) Chinese Acupuncture and Moxibustion.
〔功效〕 祛风去湿毒。
Action:Eliminating the wind toxic dampness.
〔主治〕 足癣。
Indication:Tinea pedis.
〔用法〕 电针。
Application:Electric acupuncture.

6.46.3 治癣三方
6.46.3 Prescription for The Treatment of Tinea Ⅲ

〔组成〕 曲池、然谷。
Points:Rangu(KI 2),Quchi(LI 11).
〔来源〕 宋君惠《中国针灸》1985(3)。
Source:Song Junhui 1985(3) Chinese Acupuncture and Moxibustion.
〔功效〕 补肾润肤。
Action:Reinforcing the kidney and moisturizing skin.
〔主治〕 头癣。
Indication:Tinea capitis.
〔用法〕 毫针针刺。

Application: Filiform needle acupuncture.

6.47 治牛皮癣类方
6.47 Prescriptions for Psoriasis

6.47.1 治牛皮癣一方
6.47.1 Prescription for Psoriasis I

〔组成〕 ①大椎、陶道、肝俞、脾俞;②胸5-6、腰1-2夹脊穴。
Points:(1)Dazhui(DU 14),Taodao(DU 13),Ganshu(BL 18),Pishu(BL 20);(2)Jiaji(EX-B 2, beside the 5th and 6th thoracic vertebra, and jiaji beside the 1st and 2ed lumbar vertebra).

〔来源〕 赵福蕴《北京中医》1986(2)。
Source: Zhao Fuyun 1986(2) Beijing Journal of TCM.

〔功效〕 除湿热、调营血、健脾活血止痒。
Action: Eliminating the heat and dampness, regulating the Ying (nutritive)Qi and blood;replenishing the spleen and stopping itching of skin.

〔主治〕 牛皮癣。
Indication: Psoriasis.

〔用法〕 先在第一组三棱针点刺加拔罐,后电针第2组。
Application: Apply three-edged needle pricking puncture in points of group (1);then electric acupuncture in points of group (2).

6.47.2 治牛皮癣二方
6.47.2 Prescription for Psoriasis II

〔组成〕 耳穴心、肺。
Points: Auricubar Points: Heart, Lungs.
〔来源〕 周瑞华等《辽宁中医杂志》1987(7)。
Source: Zhou Ruihua etc. 1987(7) Liaolin Journal of TCM.
〔功效〕 调营血,润肌肤。
Action: Regulating the function of Ying (nutritive) Qi and blood.
〔主治〕 牛皮癣。
Indication: Psoriasis.
〔用法〕 割治法。
Application: Apply the pricking therapy.

6.48 麦粒肿类方
6.48 Prescriptions for Hordeolum

6.48.1 麦粒肿一方
6.48.1 Prescription for Hordeolum I

〔组成〕 曲池。
Point: Quchi(LI 11)。
〔来源〕 黄国贤《四川中医》1986(4)。
Source: Huang Gouxian 1986(4) Sichuan Journal of TCM。
〔功效〕 泄热。
Action: Clearing away heat.

〔主治〕 麦粒肿。
Indication：Hordeolum.

〔用法〕 取对侧曲池点刺出血。
Application：Apply spot pricking for blood letting at the countralateral LI 11.

6.48.2 麦粒肿二方
6.48.2 Prescription for Hordeolum II

〔组成〕 后溪。
Point：Houxi(SI 3).

〔来源〕 李史光《新中医》1985(1)。
Source：Li Siguang 1985(1)New TCM Journal.

〔功效〕 疏热解毒。
Action：Clearing away heat evil and detoxication.

〔主治〕 麦粒肿。
Indication：Hordeolum.

〔用法〕 直接灸。
Application：Direct moxibustion.

6.48.3 麦粒肿三方
6.48.3 Prescription for Hordeolum III

〔组成〕 脾俞。
Point：Pishu(BL 20).

〔来源〕 《针灸秘验》。
Source：Zhen Jiu Mi Yan(The Secret Experience of Acupuncture and Moxibustion).

〔功效〕 理脾消肿。

Action: Regulating the function of the spleen and resoloving swelling.

〔主治〕 复发性麦粒肿。

Indication: Recrudescent hordeolum.

〔用法〕 艾灸。

Application: Moxibustion.

6.48.4 麦粒肿四方
6.48.4 Prescription for Hordeolum Ⅳ

〔组成〕 肝俞。

Point: Ganshu(BL 18)。

〔来源〕 吴速成、李宽厚《中国针灸》1985(3)

Source: Wu Shucheng and Li etc. 1985(3) Chinese Acupuncture and Moxibustion.

〔功效〕 调肝泄热毒。

Action: Regulating the function of liver, eliminating the toxic heat.

〔主治〕 复发性麦粒肿。

Indication: Recrudescent hordeolum.

〔用法〕 刺出血。

Application: Spot pricking for blood-letting.

6.49 目赤肿痛类方
6.49 Prescriptions for Reddish, Painful and Swollen Eye

6.49.1 目赤肿痛一方
6.49.1 Prescription for Reddish, Painful and Swollen Eye I.

〔组成〕 内迎香。
Point: Neiyinxian(EX-HN 9).

〔来源〕《扁鹊神应针灸玉龙经》。
Source: Bianque Shen Yin ZhenJiu Yu Long Jing (The Miraculous Classic of Acupucnture and Moxibustion of Bianque).

〔功效〕 疏风泄热、消肿止痛、通络明目。
Action: Dispelling the wind heat, resoloving the swelling and dredging the collaterals.

〔主治〕 目赤肿痛。
Indication: Reddish, painful and swollen eyes.

〔用法〕 刺出血。
Application: Spot pricking for blood-letting.

6.49.2 目赤肿痛二方
6.49.2 Prescription for Reddish, Painful and Swollen Eye II

〔组成〕 太阳、大骨空、小骨空。
Points: Tainyang(EX-HN 2), Dagukong(EX-UE 5), Xiaogukong

(EX-UE 6).

〔来源〕 《扁鹊神应针灸玉龙经》

Source: See 6.49.1.

〔功效〕 泄热明目。

Action: Clearing away heat and brightening the eyes.

〔主治〕 目赤肿痛。

Indication: Acute conjuctivitis.

〔用法〕 太阳刺出血,大骨空、小骨室用灸。

Application: Apply spot pricking for blood-letting in Taiyang and moxibustion in EX-UE 5 and 6.

6.49.3 目赤痛三方
6.49.3 Prescription for Reddish, Painful and Swollen Eyes III

〔组成〕 耳尖。

Points: Apex of the ear.

〔来源〕 胡宏英《中国针灸》1987(4)。

Source: Hu Hongyin 1987(4) Chinese Acupuncture and Moxibustion.

〔功效〕 清热消肿。

Action: Clearing the heat and resolving the swelling.

〔主治〕 红眼病。

Indication: Epedemic Kerato-conjuctivitis.

〔用法〕 点刺出血。

Application: Spot pricking for blood-letting.

6.50 造血系统疾病类方
6.50 Prescriptions for Disorders in Hematopoietic System

6.50.1 血液一方
6.50.1 Prescription for Disorders in Hematopoietic System Ⅰ

〔组成〕 大椎、命门、足三里。
Points: Dazhui(DU 14), Mingmen(DU 4), Zusanli(ST 36).

〔来源〕 彭正令、郭秀兰《上海针灸杂志》1986(4)。
Source: Peng Zhenling and Go Xiu Lan. 1986(4) Shanghai Journal of Acupuncture and Moxibustion.

〔功效〕 健脾益气,补肾强身,升白血球。
Action: Replenishing the kidney and spleen, increasing the quatity of leukocytes.

〔主治〕 放疗引起白细胞减少症。
Indication: Leukopenia caused by radial therapy.

〔用法〕 艾灸。
Application: Moxibustion.

6.50.2 血液二方
6.50.2 Prescription for Disorders in Hematopoietic System Ⅱ

〔组成〕 八髎、腰阳关。
Points: Baliao(BL 31, 32, 33 and 34 bilaterally) Yaoyangguang (DU 3).

〔来源〕 许美纯《新中医》1983(1)。
Source：Xu Maichun 1983(1) New Journal of TCM.

〔功效〕 补肾生髓。
Action：Reinforcing the kidney and replenishing the marrow.

〔主治〕 血小板减少症。
Indication：Thrombocytopenia.

〔用法〕 隔姜灸。
Application：Ginger slice partition indirect moxibustion.

6.51 肿瘤类方
6.51 Prescriptions for the Treatment of Tumor

6.51.1 肿瘤一方
6.51.1 Prescription for the Treatment of Tumor I

〔组成〕 子宫、曲骨、横骨、耳皮质下。
Points：Zigong(EX-CA 1), Qugu(RU 2), Henggu(KI 11), Subcortex in auricular points.

〔来源〕 王丽《中国针灸》1986(1)。
Source：Wang Li 1986(1) Chinese Acupuncture and Moxibustion.

〔功效〕 调宫活血消肿。
Action：Removing blood stasis and resolving the mass.

〔主治〕 子宫肌瘤。
Indication：Hysteromyoma.

〔用法〕 毫针针刺。
Application：Filiform needle acupuncture.

6.51.2 肿瘤二方

6.51.2 Prescription for the Treatment of Tumor Ⅱ

〔组成〕 肝炎点(右锁骨中线直下,肋弓下缘2寸处)、足三里、阳陵泉、期门、章门、三阴交。

Points: Hepatitis point: (in the right midclavicular line 2, cun below the lower border of costal arch), Zusanli(ST 36), Yanglingquan (GB 34), Qimen(LR 14), Zhangmen(LR 13), Sanyinjiao (SP 6).

〔来源〕 熊裕家《湖北中医杂志》1986(6)。

Source: Xiong Yujia, 1986(6) Hubai Journal of TCM.

〔功效〕 调肝止痛。

Action: Regulating the function of the liver and relieving pain.

〔主治〕 肝癌疼痛。

Indication: Hepatalgia in patient with liver cancer.

〔用法〕 毫针针刺。

Application: Filiform needle acupuncture.

6.51.3 肿瘤三方

6.51.3 Prescription for The Treatment of Tumor Ⅲ

〔组成〕 孔最、阿是。

Pionts: Kongzhui(LU 6), Ashi pionts.

〔来源〕 左秀玲验方。

Source: Zuo Xiuling's experience.

〔功效〕 宣肺止痛。

Action: Disperssing the stagnant Qi in lungs and relieving the pain.

〔主治〕 肺癌疼痛。

Indication: The pain of patient with lung cancer.

〔用法〕 毫针强刺激,留针 30~60 分钟。

Application: Apply intense stimulation with filiform needle, retain the needle for 30-60 minutes.

附录 I 针灸穴位索引表

APPENDIX ONE CROSS INDEX OF ACUPOINTS

B

Bafeng 八风(EX—LE 10)

Baichongwu 百虫窝(EX—LE 3)

Baihuanshu 白环俞(BL 30)

Baihui 百会(DU 20)

Baohuang 胞肓(BL 53)

Baxie 八邪(EX—UE 9)

Benshen 本神(GB 13)

Biguan 髀关(ST 31)

Binao 臂臑(LI 14)

Bingfeng 秉风(SI 12)

Bulang 步廊(KI 22)

Burong 不容(ST 19)

C

Changqiang 长强(DU 1)
Chengfu 承扶(BL 36)
Chengguang 承光(BL 6)
Chengjiang 承浆(RN 24)
Chengjin 承筋(BL 56)
Chengling 承灵(GB 18)
Chengman 承满(ST 20)
Chengqi 承泣(ST 1)
Chengshan 承山(BL 57)
chize 尺泽(LU 5)
Chongmen 冲门(SP 12)
Chimai 瘛脉(SJ 18)
Chongyang 冲阳(ST 42)
Ciliao 次髎(BL 32)
Cuanzhu 攒竹(BL 2)

D

Dabao 大包(SP 21)
Dachangshu 大肠俞(BL 25)
Dadu 大都 SP 2)
Dadun 大敦(LR 1)
Dagukong 大骨空(EX—UE 5)
Dahe 大赫(KI 12)
Daheng 大横(SP 15)
Daimai 带脉(GB 26)
Daju 大巨(ST 27)

Daling 大陵(PC 7)
Dannang 胆囊穴(EX—LE 6)
Danshu 胆俞(BL 19)
Dangyang 当阳(EX—HN 2)
Dazhu 大杼(BL 11)
Daying 大迎(ST 5)
Dazhong 大钟(KI 4)
Dazhui 大椎(DU 14)
Dicang 地仓(ST 4)
Diji 地机(SP 8)
Dingchuan 定喘(EX—B 1)
Diwuhui 地五会(GB 42)
Duiduan 兑端(DU 27)
Dubi 犊鼻(ST 35)
Dushu 督俞(BL 16)
Duyin 独阴(EX—LE 11)

E

Erbai 二白(EX—UE 2)
Erjian 二间(LI 2)
Erjian 耳尖(EX—HN 6)
Ermen 耳门(SJ 21)

F

Feishu 肺俞(BL 13)
Feiyang 飞扬(BL 58)
Fengchi 风池(GB 20)

Fengfu 风府(DU 16)
Fenglong 丰隆(ST 40)
Fengmen 风门(BL 12)
Fengshi 风市(GB 31)
Fuai 腹哀(SP 16)
Fubai 浮白(GB 10)
Fufen 附分(BL 41)
Fujie 腹结(SP 14)
Fuliu 复溜(KI 7)
Fushe 府舍(SP 13)
Futonggu 腹通谷(KI 20)
Futu 扶突(LI 18)
Futu 伏兔(ST 32)
Fuyang 跗阳(BL 59)
Fuxi 浮郄(BL 38)

G

Ganshu 肝俞(BL 18)
Gaohuang 膏肓(BL 43)
Geguan 膈关(BL 46)
Geshu 膈俞(BL 17)
Gongsun 公孙(SP 4)
Guanchong 关冲(SJ 1)
Guangming 光明(GB 37)
Guanmen 关门(ST 22)
Guanyuan 关元(RN 4)
Guanyuanshu 关元俞(BL 26)
Guilai 归来(ST 29)

H

Hanyan 颔厌(GB 4)
Haiquan 海泉(EX—HN 11)
Heding 鹤顶(EX—LE2)
Hegu 合谷(LI 4)
Heliao 和髎(SJ 22)
Henggu 横骨(KI 11)
Heyang 合阳(BL 55)
Houding 后顶(DU 19)
Houxi 后溪(SI 3)
Huagai 华盖(BN 20)
Huangmen 肓门(BL 51)
Huangshu 肓俞(KI 16)
Huantiao 环跳(GB 30)
Hunmen 魂门(BL 47)
Huaroumen 滑肉门(ST 24)
Huiyang 会阳(BL 35)
Huiyin 会阴(RN 1)
Huizong 会宗(SJ 7)
Hunmen 魂门(BL 47)

J

Jiache 颊车(ST 6)
Jiaji 夹脊(EX—B 2)
Jianjing 肩井(GB 21)
Jianli 建里(RN 11)
Jianliao 肩髎(SJ 14)

Jianshi 间使(PC 5)

Jianwaishu 肩外俞(SI 14)

Jianyu 肩髃(LI 15)

Jianzhen 肩贞(SI 9)

Jianzhongshu 肩中俞(SI 15)

Jiaosun 角孙(SJ 20)

Jiaoxin 交信(KI 8)

Jiexi 解溪(ST 41)

Jimai 急脉(LR 12)

Jimen 箕门(SP 11)

Jinggu 京骨(BL 64)

Jingbailao 颈百劳(EX—HN 15)

Jingmen 京门(GB25)

Jingming 睛明(BL 1)

Jinqu 经渠(LU 8)

Jinjin 金津(EX—HN 12)

Jinmen 金门(BL 63)

Jinsuo 筋缩(DU 8)

Jiquan 极泉(HT 1)

Jiuwei 鸠尾(RN 15)

Jizhong 脊中(DU 6)

Juegu 绝骨(GB 39)

Jueyinshu 厥阴俞(BL 14)

Jugu 巨骨(LI 16)

Juliao 巨髎(ST 3)

Juliao 居髎(GB 29)

Juquan 聚泉(EX—HN 10)

Juque 巨阙(RN 14)

K

Kongzui 孔最(LU 6)
Kouheliao 禾髎(LI 19)
Kuangu 髋骨(EX—LE 1)
Kufang 库房(ST 14)
Kunlun 昆仑(BL 60)

L

Lanwei 阑尾穴(EX—LE 7)
Laogong 劳宫(PC 8)
Liangmen 梁门(ST 21)
Liangqiu 梁丘(ST 34)
Lianquan 廉泉(RN 23)
Liduii 厉兑(ST 45)
Lieque 列缺(LU 7)
Ligou 蠡沟(LR 5)
Lingdao 灵道(HT 4)
Lingtai 灵台(DU 10)
Lingxu 灵墟(KI 24)
Lougu 漏谷(SP 7)
Luoque 络却(BL 8)
Luxi 颅息(SJ 19)

M

Meichong 眉冲(BL 3)
Mingmen 命门(DU 4)

Muchuang 目窗(GB 16)

N

Naohu 脑户(DU 17)
Naohui 臑会(SJ 13)
Naokong 脑空(GB 19)
Naoshu 臑俞(SJ 10)
Neiguan 内关(PC 6)
Neihuaijian 内踝尖(EX—LE 8)
Neixiyan 内膝眼(EX—LE 4)
Neiyingxiang 内迎香(EX—HN 9)
Neiting 内庭(ST 44)

P

Pangguangshu 膀胱俞(BL 28)
Pianli 偏历(LI 6)
Pigen 痞根(EX—B 4)
Pishu 脾俞(BL 20)
Pohu 魄户(BL 42)
Pushen 仆参(BL 61)

Q

Qianding 前顶(DU 21)
Qiangjian 强间(DU 18)
Qiangu 前谷(SI 2)
Qichong 气冲(ST 30)
Qiduan 气端(EX—LE 12)

409

Qihai 气海(RN 6)
Qihaishu 气海俞(BL 24)
Qihu 气户(ST 13)
Qimai 瘈脉(SJ 18)
Qimen 期门(LR 14)
Qinglengyuan 清冷渊(SJ 11)
Qingling 青灵(HT 2)
Qishe 气舍(ST 11)
Qiuhou 球后(EX—HN 7)
Qiuxu 丘墟(GB 40)
Qixue 气穴(KI 13)
Quanliao 颧髎(SI 18)
Qubin 曲鬓(GB 7)
Quchai 曲差(BL 4)
Quchi 曲池(LI 11)
Quepen 缺盆(ST 12)
Qugu 曲骨(RN 2)
Ququan 曲泉(LR 8)
Quyuan 曲垣(SI 13)
Quze 曲泽(PC 3)

R

Rangu 然谷(KI 2)
Renying 人迎(ST 9)
Renzhong 人中(DU 26)
Riyue 日月(GB 24)
Rugen 乳根(ST 18)
Ruzhong 乳中(ST 17)

S

Sanjian 三间(LI 3)

Sanjiaoshu 三焦俞(BL 22)

Sanyanluo 三阳络(SJ 8)

Sanyinjiao 三阴交(SP 6)

Shangguan 上关(GB 3)

Shangjuxu 上巨虚(ST 37)

Shanglian 上廉(LI 9)

Shangliao 上髎(BL 31)

Shangqiu 商丘(SP 5)

Shangqu 商曲(KI 17)

Shangwan 上脘(RN 13)

Shangxin 上星(DU 23)

Shangyingxiang 上迎香(EX—HN 8)

Shangyang 商阳(LI 1)

Shaochong 少冲(HT 9)

Shaofu 少府(HT 8)

Shaohai 少海(HT 3)

Shaoshang 少商(LU 11)

Shaoze 少泽(SI 1)

Shencang 神藏(KI 25)

Shendao 神道(DU 11)

Shenfeng 神封(KI 23)

Shenque 神阙(RN 8)

Shenmai 申脉(BL 62)

Shenshu 肾俞(BL 23)

Shentang 神堂(BL 44)

Shenting 神庭(DU 24)
Shenzhu 身柱(DU 12)
Shidou 食窦(SP 17)
Shiguan 石关(KI 18)
Shimen 石门(RN 5)
Shiqizhui 十七椎(EX—B 8)
Shixuan 十宣(EX—UE 11)
Shousanli 手三里(LI 10)
Shouwuli 手五里(LI 13)
Shuaigu 率谷(GB 8)
Shugu 束骨(BL 65)
Shufu 俞府(KI 27)
Shuidao 水道(ST 38)
Shuifen 水分(RN 9)
Shuigou 水沟(DU 26)
Shuiquan 水泉(KI 5)
Shuitu 水突(ST 10)
Sibai 四白(ST 2)
Sidu 四渎(SJ 9)
Sifeng 四缝(EX—UE 10)
Siman 四满(KI 14)
Sishencong 四神聪(EX-HN 1)
Sizhukong 丝竹空(SJ 23)
Suliao 素髎(DU 25)

T

Taibai 太白(SP 3)
Taichong 太冲(LR 3)

Taixi 太溪(KI 3)
Taiyang 太阳(EX—HN 15)
TaiYi 太乙(ST 23)
Taiyuan 太渊(LU 9)
Tanzhong 膻中(RN 17)
Taodao 陶道(DU 13)
Tianchi 天池(PC 1)
Tianchong 天冲(GB 9)
Tianchuang 天窗(SI 16)
Tianding 天鼎(LI 17)
Tianfu 天府(LU 3)
Tianjing 天井(SJ 10)
Tianliao 天髎(SJ 15))
Tianquan 天泉(PC 2)
Tianrong 天容(SI 17)
Tianshu 天枢(ST 25)
Tiantu 天突(RN 22)
Tianxi 天溪(SP 18)
Tianyou 天牖(SJ 16)
Tianzhu 天柱(BL 10)
Tianzong 天宗(SI 11)
Tiaokou 条口(ST 38)
Tinggong 听宫(SI 19)
Tinghui 听会(GB 2)
Tongli 通里(HT 5)
Tongtian 通天(BL 7)
Tongziliao 瞳子髎(GB 1)
Toulinqi 头临泣(GB 15)

413

Touqiaoyin 头窍阴(GB 11)
Touwei 头维(ST 8)

W

Waiguan 外关(SJ 5)
Wailing 外陵(ST 26)
Waihuaijian 外踝尖(EX—LE 9)
Wailaogong 外劳宫(EX—UE 8)
Waiqui 外丘(GB 36)
Wangu 完骨(GB 12)
Wangu 腕骨(SI 4)
Weicang 胃仓(BL 50)
Weidao 维道(GB 28)
Weiwanxiashu 胃脘下俞(EX—B 3)
Weishu 胃俞(BL 21)
Weiyang 委阳(BL.39)
Weizhong 委中(BL 40)
Wenliu 温溜(LI 7)
Wuchu 五处(BL 5)
Wushu 五枢(GB 27)
Wuyi 屋翳(ST 15)

X

Xiguan 膝关(LR 7)
Xiyan 膝眼(EX—LE 5)
Xiyangguan 膝阳关(GB 33)
Xiaguan 下关(ST 7)

Xiajishu 下极俞(EX－B 5)

Xiajuxu 下巨虚(ST 39)

Xialian 下廉(LI 8)

Xialiao 下髎(BL 34)

Xiaogukong 小骨空(EX－UE 6)

Xiaxi 侠溪(GB 43)

Xiabai 侠白(LU 4)

Xiawan 下脘(RN 10)

Ximen 郄门(PC 4)

Xiangu 陷谷(ST 43)

Xiaochangshu 小肠俞(BL 27)

Xiaohai 小海(SI 8)

Xiaoluo 消泺(SJ 12)

Xingjian 行间(LR 2)

Xinhui 囟会(DU 22)

Xinshu 心俞(BL 15)

Xiongxiang 胸乡(SP 19)

Xuanji 璇玑(RN 21)

Xuanli 悬厘(GB 6)

Xuanlu 悬颅(GB 5)

Xuanshu 悬枢(DU 5)

Xuanzhong 悬钟(GB 39)

Xuehai 血海(SP 10)

Y

Yamen 哑门(DU 15)

Yangbai 阳白(GB 14)

Yangchi 阳池(SJ 4)

Yangfu 阳辅(GB 38)
Yanggang 阳纲(BL 48)
Yanggu 阳谷(SI 5)
Yangjiao 阳交(GB 35)
Yanglao 养老(SI 6)
Yanglingquan 阳陵泉(GB 34)
Yangxi 阳溪(LI 5)
Yaoqi 腰奇(EX—B 9)
Yaoshu 腰俞(DU 2)
Yaotongdian 腰痛点(EX—UE 7)
Yaoyan 腰眼(EX—B 7)
Yaoyangguan 腰阳关(DU 3)
Yaoyi 腰宜(EX—B 6)
Yemen 液门(SJ 2)
Yifeng 翳风(SJ 17)
Yiming 翳明(EX—HN 14)
Yinbai 隐白(SP 1)
Yinbao 阴包(LR 9)
Yindu 阴都(KI 19)
Yingchuang 膺窗(ST 16)
Yingu 阴谷(KI 10)
Yingxiang 迎香(LI 20)
Yinjiao 阴交(RN 7)
Yinjiao 龈交(DU 28)
Yinlian 阴廉(LR 11)
Yinlingquan 阴陵泉(SP 9)
Yinmen 殷门(BL 37)
Yinshi 阴市(ST 33)

Yintang 印堂(EX—HN 3)
Yinxi 阴郄(HT 6)
Yishe 意舍(BL 49)
Yixi 譩譆(BL 45)
Yongquan 涌泉(KI 1)
Youmen 幽门(KI 21)
Yuanye 渊腋(GB 22)
Yuji 鱼际(LU 10)
Yunmen 云门(LU 2)
Yutang 玉堂(RN 18)
Yuyao 鱼腰(EX—HN 4)
Yuye 玉液(EX—HN 13)
Yuzhen 玉枕(BL 9)
Yuzhong 彧中(KI 26)

Z

Zanzhu 攒竹(BL 2)
Zhangmen 章门(LR 13)
Zhaohai 照海(KI 6)
Zhejin 辄筋(GB 23)
Zhengying 正营(GB 17)
Zhibian 秩边(BL 54)
Zhigou 支沟(SJ 6)
Zhishi 志室(BL 52)
Zhiyang 至阳(DU 9)
Zhiyin 至阴(BL 67)
Zhizheng 支正(SI 7)
Zhongchong 中冲(PC 9)

Zhongdu 中渎(GB 32)
Zhongdu 中都(LR 6)
Zhongfeng 中封(LR 4)
Zhongfu 中府(LU 1)
Zhongji 中极(RN 3)
Zhongkui 中魁(EX—UE 4)
Zhonglushu 中膂俞(BL 29)
Zhongquan 中泉(EX—UE 3)
Zhongshu 中枢(DU 7)
Zhongting 中庭(RN 16)
Zhongwan 中脘(RN 12)
Zhongzhu 中注(KI 15)
Zhongzhu 中渚(SJ 3)
Zhoujian 肘尖(EX—UE 1)
Zhouliao 肘髎(LI 12)
Zhourong 周荣(SP 20)
Zhubin 筑宾(KI 9)
Zigong 紫宫(RN 19)
Zigong 子宫(EX—CA 1)
Zulinqi 足临泣(GB 41)
Zuqiaoyin 足窍阴(GB 44)
Zusanli 足三里(ST 36)
Zutonggu 足通谷(BL 66)
Zuwuli 足五里(LR 10)

附录 Ⅱ 经外奇穴的定位
APPENDIX TWO THE LOCATIONS OF EXTRA-ACUPOINTS

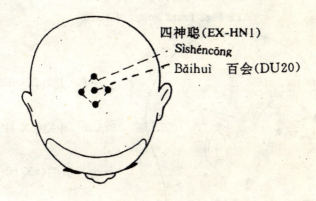

附图 1 四神聪穴
App Fig1 Sishencong (EX-HN 1)

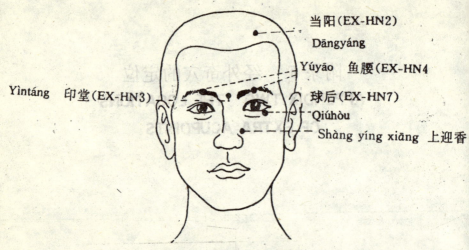

附图2 经外穴(头面部)
APP Fig2 Extra Points of Head

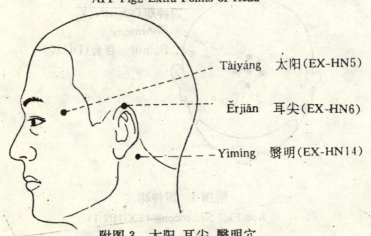

附图3 太阳、耳尖、翳明穴
App Fig3 Taiyang (EX-HN 5), Erjian(EX-HN6) and Yiming(EX—HN14)

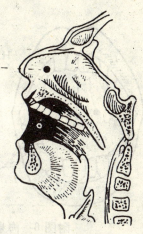

附图4 内迎香穴
App Fig 4 Neiyingxiang (EX-HN9)

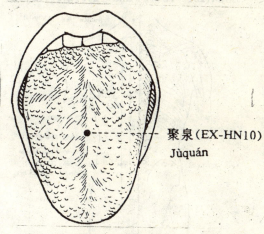

附图5 聚泉穴
App Fig5 Juquan(EX-HN10)

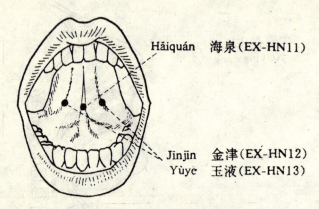

附图6 海泉、金津、玉液穴
App Fig6 Haiquan(EX—HN11), Jinjin(EX—HN12) and Yuye(EX—HN13)

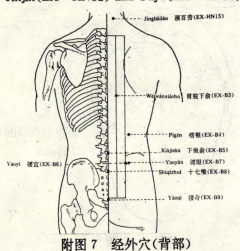

附图7 经外穴(背部)
App Fig7 Extra Points on Back

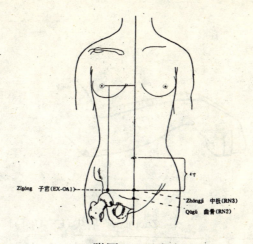

附图8 子宫穴
App Fig8 Zigong(EX—CA1)

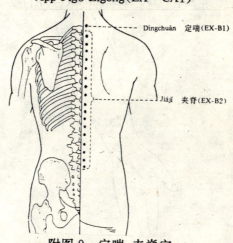

附图9 定喘、夹脊穴
App Fig9 Dingchuan(EX—B1) and Jiaji (EX—B2)

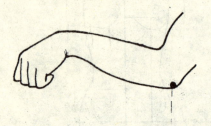

Zhōujiān 肘尖(EX-UE1)

附图10 肘尖穴
App Fig10 Zhoujian(EX—UE1)

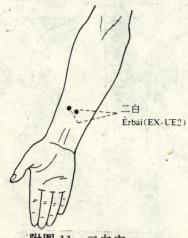

二白
Èrbái(EX-UE2)

附图11 二白穴
App Fig11 Erbai(EX—UE2)

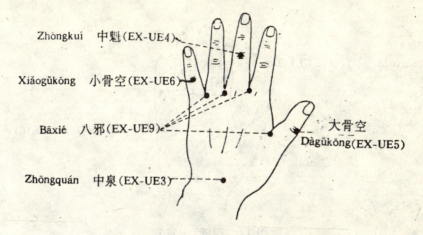

附图 12　经外穴(手背)
App Fig12 Extra Points (Dorsum of Hand)

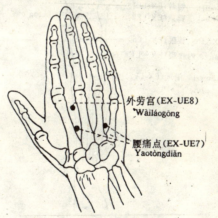

附图 13　腰痛点、外劳宫穴
App Fig13 Yaotongdian(Ex—UE7)and Wailaogong(EX—UE8)

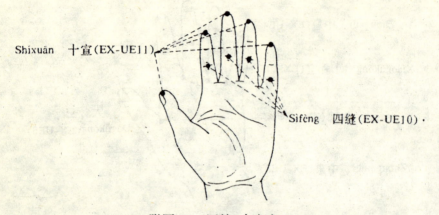

附图 14 四缝、十宣穴
App Fig14 Sifeng(EX—UE10) and Shixuan (EX—UE11)

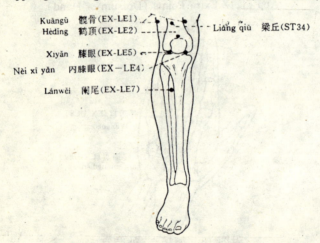

附图 15 髋骨、鹤顶、膝眼、阑尾穴
App Fig15 Kuangu(EX—LE1),Heding (EX—LE2)
Xiyan(EX—LE5) and Lanwei (EX—LE7)

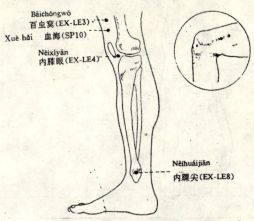

附图 16 百虫窝、内膝眼、内踝尖穴
App Fig16 Baichongwo (EX—LE3),
Neixiyan (EX—LE4) and Neihuaijian (EX—LE8)

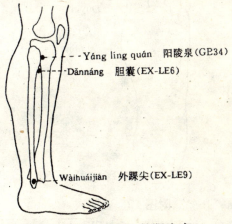

附图 17 胆囊、外踝尖穴
App Fig17 Dannang (EX—LE6) and
Weihuaijian (EX—LE9)

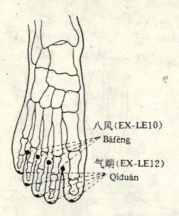

附图 18 八风、气端穴
App Fig18 Bafeng (EX—LE10) and Qiduan(EX—LE12)

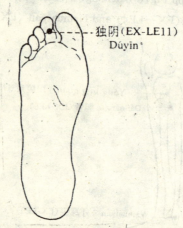

附图 19 独阴穴
App Fig19 Duyin (EX—LE11)

附录 Ⅲ 参考文献
APPENDIX THREE THE BILIOGRAPHY

1. Bianque Xin Shu (The Secret Book of Bianque) By Dou Cai, Song Dynasty (扁鹊心书,宋·窦材)

2. Bai Zhen Fu (The Poems of Acupuncture Treatment of Syndromes) by Gao Wu, Ming Dynasty. *The Book is part of the Zhen Jiu Ju Yin (The Essence of Acupuncture and Moxibustion)*

(百症赋,明·高武,该书是针灸聚英的一部分)

3. Chong Lou Yu Yao (The Jade Key of Medical Mansion) by Zheng Mei Jian, Qing Dynasty (重楼玉钥,清·郑梅涧)

4. Gu Jin Yi Tiong (The General Medicine of Past and Present), by Xu Chun Fu, Ming Dynasty (古今医统,明·徐春甫)

5. Er Zhen Zhen Zhi Fa (The Diagnostic and Therapeutic Techniques of Auricular Acupuncture) by Li Zhi Ming, Ancient Traditional Chinese Medical Literature Press, 1988. (耳针诊治法·李志明,中医古籍出版社,1988)

6. Jiu Fa Mi Zhuan (The Secret Teaching in Moxibustion) by Lei Shao Yi, Qing Dynasty (灸法秘传,清·雷少逸)

7. Jin Gui Gou Xian (The Gist of Golden Chamber) by Zu Dan Xi, Yuan Dynasty (金匮钩玄,元·朱丹溪)

8. Jing Yue Quan Shu (Jingyue's Complete Works) by Zhang Jing Yue, Ming Dynasty (景岳全书,明·张景岳)

9. Nei Jing Zhen Jiu Lei Fang Yu Si (The Explanation of Acupuncture Prescriptions in Nei Jing) by Zhang Shuan Chen, Shangdon Science and Technology Press, 1980(内经针灸类方语释,张善忱,山东科技出版社,1980)

10. Qian Jin Fang (The Valuable Prescriptions) by Sun Si Miao, Tang Dynasty (千金方·唐·孙思邈)

11. Qian Zhai Jian Xia Lian Fang (The Simple and Effective Prescriptions From The Sceret Room) by Wang Shi Xiong, Qing Dynasty (千金简效良方,清·王士雄)

12. Pi Wei Lun (The Treatise Of Spleen and Stomach) by Li Gao, Jin Dynasty(脾胃论,金·李杲)

13. Pu Ji Fang (The Prescriptions for Curing All People), Zhu Shu et al, eds, Ming Dynasty(普济方,明·朱橚等编撰)

14. Lu Shou Yan Zhen Jiu Lun Zhu Yi An Xian (The Selection of Works and Cases Treated With Acupuncture and Moxibustion by Lu Shou Yan) by Wu Shao De, People's Health Press, 1984(陆瘦燕针灸论著医案选,吴绍德,人民卫生出版社,1984)

15. Ru Men Shi Qin (Prerequisite Knowledge for Physicians) by Zhang Zi He, Jin Dynasty (儒门事亲,金·张子和)

16. Shou Zhen Xin Liao Fa (New Technique of Hand—Acupoint Acupuncture) by Zhu Zhen Hua, Peoples Army Medical Press, 1990 (手针新疗法,朱振华,人民军医出版社,1990)

17. Shen Jiu Jing Lun (The Protocol of Miraculous Moxibustion) by Wu Yi Ding, Qing Dynasty(神灸经纶,清·吴亦鼎)

18. Wai Tai Mi Yao (The Necessities of a Frontier Official) by Wang Tao, Tang Dynasty (752 AD.)(外台秘要,唐·王焘)

19. Yi Wue Zhen Zhuan (The Orthodox Medical Record) by Yu Tian Ming, Ming Dynasty(医学正传,明·虞天民)

20. Yan Zhen Liao Fa (The Eye Acupuncture) by Peng Jing Shan, Liaoning Science and Technology Press. 1990(眼针疗法,彭静山,辽宁科技出版社,1990)

21. Yi Xue Gang Mu (The Outling of Medicine) by Lou Ying, Ming Dynasty(医学纲目,明·楼英)

22. Yu Long Jing (The Classic of Jade Dragon) by Wang Guo Rui, Yuan Dynasty(玉龙经,元·王国瑞)

23. Yi Zong Jin Jian (The Golden Mirror of Medicine) by Wu Qian, Qing Dynasty(医宗金鉴,清·吴谦)

24. Yi Shuo (The Explanation of Medicine) by Zhang Gao, Song Dynasty(医说,宋·张杲)

25. Zhen Jin Mi Yan (The Secret Experience in Acupuncture and Moxibustion) By Pen Jing Shan, Liaoning Science and Technology Press,1985(针灸秘验,彭静山,辽宁科技出版社,1985)

26. Zhen Jiu Da Cheng (The Great Compendium of Acupuncture and Moxibustion) by Yang Ji Zhou, Ming Dynasty(针灸大成,明·杨继州)

27. Zhen Jiu Da Qian (The Complete Works of Acupuncture and Moxibustion) by Xu Feng, Ming Dynasty(针灸大全,明·徐凤)

28. Zhen Jiu Ji Cheng (The Collected Works of Acupuncture and Moxibustion) by Liao Run Hong, Qing Dynasty (针灸集成,清·廖润鸿)

29. Zhen Jiu Zi Nan (The Classic of Acupuncture Act as Compasses) by Dou Han Qing, Jing Dynasty(针经指南,金元·窦汉卿)

30. Zhen Jiu Zhen Zong (The Orthodox Record of Acupuncture and Moxibustion) by Lu Shao Yan, Shanghai New Chinese Institute of Acup. and Moxib. Press, 1950(针灸正宗,陆瘦燕,上海新中国针灸研究出版社出版,1950)

31. Zhen Jiu Feng Yuan (The Origin of Acupuncture and Moxibustion) by Li Xue Chuang, Qing Dynasty (针灸逢源,清·李学川)

32. Za Bin Xue Fa Ge (The Poems of Acupuncture Treatment of Internal Diseases) by Li Chan, Ming Dynasty. *The book is part of Yi Xue Ru Men (Elementary Course of Medicine) by Li Chan* (杂病穴法歌,明·李梴,该书为医学入门的一部分)

33. Zhen Fang Liu Ji (The Six Chapters of Acupucnture Prescriptions) by Wu Kun, Ming Dynasty(针方六集,明·吴昆)

34. Zhen Jiu Ja Yi Jing Jiao Si (The AB Classic of Acupuncture and Moxibustion with Annotations) Shandong College of TCM eds, People's Health Press, 1957(针灸甲乙经校释,山东中医学院编,人民卫生出版社,1957)

35. Zhen Jiu Zi Shen Jing (The Classic of Curing People With Acupuncture and Moxibustion) by Wang Zhi Zhong, Song Dynasty(针灸资生经,宋·王执中)

36. Zhen Jiu Ju Ying (Essence of Experience of the Eminent Aupuncturists) by Gao Wu, Ming Dynasty(针灸聚英,明·高武)

37. Zhen Jiu Lin Zheng Zhi Nan (The Handbook for Clinic Practice of Acupuncture and Moxibustion) by Hu Xi Ming et al, eds, People's Health Press, 1991(针灸临证指南,胡熙明等,人民卫生出版社,1991)

38. Zhong Yi Zhen Fa Ji jing (The Collecton of Acupuncture Techniques) by Liu Guan Jun, Jiangxi Science and Technology Press, 1988(中医针法集锦,刘冠军,江西科技出版社,1988)

39. Zhong·Yi Fu Ke Xue (Gynecology of Traditional Chinese medicine), Hubai College of TCM eds, Shanghai Science and Technology Press, 1980 (中医妇科学,湖北中医学院编,上海科技出版社,1980)

40. Zhong Guo Zhen Jiu Chu Fang Xue (Chinese Acupuncture and Moxibustion Prescriptions) by Xiao Shao Qin, Ningxia People's Health Press, 1986(中国针灸处方学,肖少卿,宁夏人民卫生出版社,1986)

41. Tong Ren Su Xue Zhen Jiu Tu Jing (The Illustrated Manual on the Points for Acupuncture and Moxibustion as Found on the Bronze Figure) by Wang Wei Yi, Song Dynasty(铜人腧穴针灸图经,宋·王惟一)

42. Zhen Jui Xue (Acupuncture and Moxibustion) by Qiu Mao Lian eds, Shanghai Science and Technology Press, 1985(针灸学,邱茂良主编,上海科技出版社,1985)

43. Zhui Jia Shi Jian Zhen Jiu Fa (The Optimum Time for Acupuncture) by Liu Bing Quan, Shandong Science and Technology Press, 1988

(最佳时间治疗学,刘炳权,山东科技出版社,1988)

(赣)新登字第003号

汉英针灸治疗手册
谢金华等　编著
江西科学技术出版社出版发行
(南昌市新魏路)
各地新华书店经销　南昌市光华印刷厂印刷
开本 850×1168　1/32　印张 14.125　字数 37 万
1994 年 12 月第 1 版　1994 年 12 月第 1 次印刷
印数 1—4,000
ISBN7—5390—0779—6/R·180　定价：15.00元
(江西科技版图书凡属印刷、装订错误,请随时向承印厂调换)